GOLF

THE NEW TESTAMENT

Novus Plus GmbH Publishing Company
Carl Benz Str. 6
75217 Birkenfeld / Germany

Published in August 2012 by
Novus Plus GmbH Publishing Company

Editorial Department:
Daniel Kurz, Stephanie Valdemar, Cornelia John

Photos:
Rüdiger Schulz, F1 Online

Layout:
Bastian Uhlending

Composition:
Bastian Uhlending

Art Director:
Andrea Drollinger

Printed in Germany:
ISBN 978-3-9405-5619-6
1st edition

Think different.

«Here's to the crazy ones. The misfits. The rebels. The troublemakers. The round pegs in the square holes. The ones who see things differently. They're not fond of rules. And they have no respect for the status quo. ... They push the human race forward.»

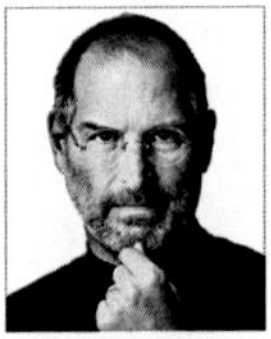

Steve Jobs
Apple founder
(1955 - 2011)

GOLF: THE NEW TESTAMENT

Foreword

Golf is a fascinating and exciting sport. Anyone who has grasped the passion for this sport wants one thing above all:

„To constantly improve their game without being injured in doing so."

Trust me when I say that you will achieve this goal with the Golf Active Method FREE-RELEASE® (GAM FREE-RELEASE®) I have developed.

The GAM FREE-RELEASE® provides you with a methodical tool for a biomechanically optimal golf swing.

On the following pages I will show you – comprehensibly and clearly – how to use this tool. The central elements of the GAM FREE-RELEASE® are described in five main instructions, called the 5 Easy Upgrades, so that in future you will have a simple plan for your swing that is applicable in any situation. With this checklist you will be able to achieve a high repeatability rate of consistent strokes.

Golfers often have an above-average educational background and good professional qualifications.

As decision-makers, many golfers are accustomed to making decisions on the basis of presentations prepared by professionally qualified employees. I have also taken this precise path in the development of GAM FREE-RELEASE®.

That is why all of my technical statements and the efficiency of GAM FREE-RELEASE® are documented through precisely measured facts.

Regardless of whether you are a captain of industry, a housewife or competitive athlete; in golf you should trust only objectively ascertained facts.

During the ten-year developmental process for GAM FREE-RELEASE®, I was always guided by the working principle of measureable results.

I wish you lasting enjoyment in the game. You should also take advantage of the chance to make a qualified decision about the choice of swing technique based on objective facts.

Ask your instructor how the stress on your body affects his or her teaching method. The handicap which you have today does not play a role in this connection.

You will improve four times faster with the GAM FREE-RELEASE®. The motion sequence of the golf swing will also be simplified by a factor of 4 and you will reduce your risk of injury by a factor of 15 with my modern method and the associated hardware.

GOLF: THE NEW TESTAMENT is the first genuinely new teaching method since the great Ben Hogan.

It leads the golfing world in terms of physiology and energy transfer.

GAM FREE-RELEASE® is the new control technique in the realm of golf.

Best regards,
Frank Drollinger

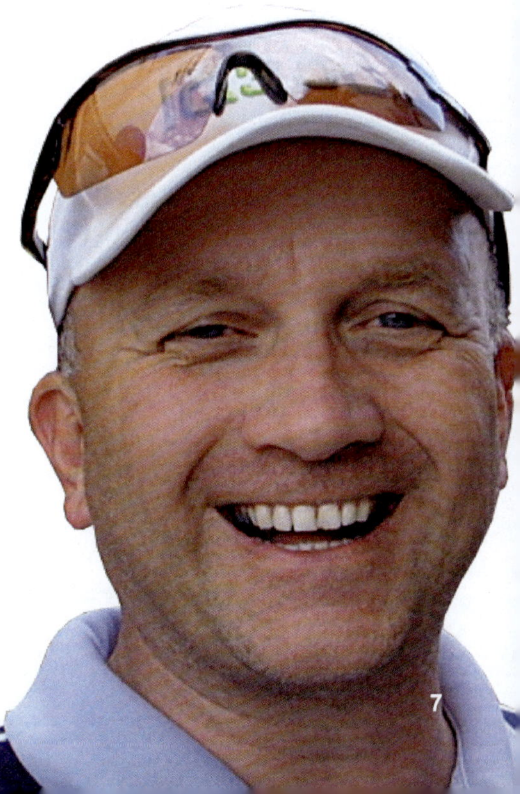

Table of Contents

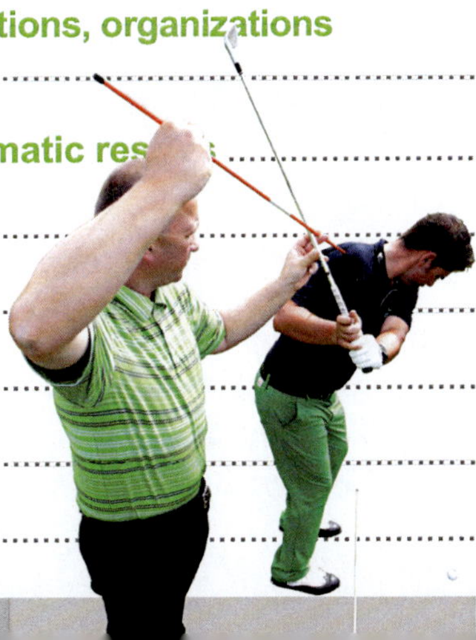

Golf-Myths

Myth 1

"You will not suffer injuries provided you execute the golf swing correctly using the existing swing method."

Not true: The strain and forces amount to 15 times the body weight where the existing swing method is correctly executed, e.g. by Tiger Woods and Rory McIlroy. This strain is reduced by up to 99% where the method developed by Frank Drollinger is used.

Myth 2

"Turning your left foot out reduces the forces affecting the body so that I no longer suffer injuries."

Not true: All tour pros who turn out their left foot suffer from injuries. In addition, turning out the left foot results in vertical torsion. The consequences adversely affect the target precision.

Myth 3

"Spikeless shoes help to reduce torsion."

Not true: A spikeless shoe the sole of which grips the turf cannot turn functionally. This recommendation is also very dangerous on slopes since you can slip if your stance is unstable.

Myth 4

"Spikeless pimple out-soles reduce torsion."

Not true: Two pimples form an axis, e.g. 60 pimples form 3,540 axes. This means that a shoe with a pimple out-sole cannot turn functionally, like studded shoes or cleats. The Turning Shoe alone turns functionally.

Myth 5

"A golf ball hit with the clubface can still be influenced after the moment of impact."

Not true: After the ball has been hit, its flight trajectory can no longer be influenced by the golfer. (proven by Dr.-Ing., Dipl.-Phys. Johannes Bertsch)

Myth 6

"The additional rules owing to the Olympic Games do not apply until 2016."

Not true: The new rules have to be applied in training and competition as of the date of application for the Olympic Games (2008). This means that every effort has to be made to minimize the risk of injury.

Myth 7

"If the turn is triggered by a slight impulse from the middle to the right, the body's center of gravity will shift approx. 3 cm to the right."

Not true: Where there is an impulse to the right, 85% of the body weight will shift to the back foot. This means that the center of gravity will shift approx. 15 cm to the right. This has been proven by measurements using foot pressure plates.

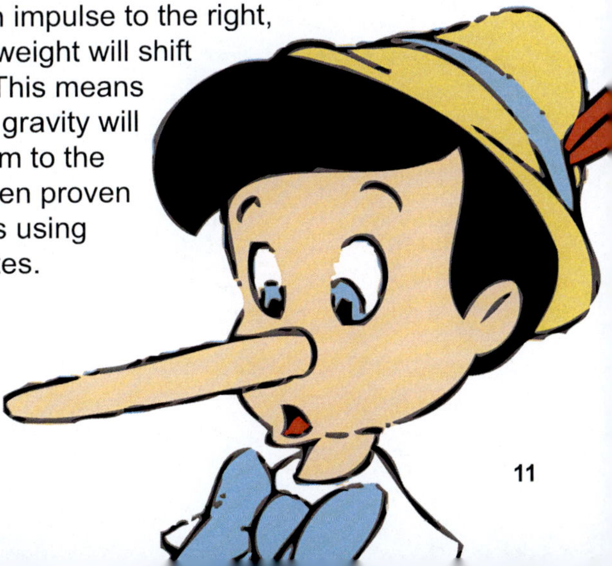

Greetings from
Dr. med. Hans-Christoph Bosch

In an era where medical and sports specialists put traditional approaches to the test with increasingly precise scientific methods, align prevention as well as therapy to the results of scientific studies, evaluate training methods and athletic techniques as well as competition schedules by means of scientific data and only acknowledge new methods if they meet these scientific requirements, it may seem surprising that the golf swing characterized by Ben Hogan (1912-1997) is still practiced purely intuitively throughout the world.

At the same time, current research shows that the golf swing is by no means a motion sequence that is particularly beneficial to health.

It is an important time to critically scrutinize and question this sport's technique.

The interesting studies by Prof. Dr. Wank (Tübingen, Germany) – who was able to ascertain an immense reduction in harmful torsional forces affecting the musculoskeletal system during a golf swing when the FREE-RELEASE® Shoe (Turning Shoe) is worn in comparison with a conventional golf shoe – have been impressively confirmed through the data recently published by the American television channel ESPN. According to this data, torsional and braking forces on the left knee exceeding 15 times the body weight have greatly affected Tiger Woods (max. club head speed over 200 km/h; 1,400°/sec.; centripetal force over 45 kg). With his weight of approx. 84 kg, this is roughly equal to 1,260 kg of force.

Therefore it may not be surprising that this leads to serious damage such as fatigue fractures of the tibial plateau.

Based on a solid scientific basis of data, Frank Drollinger has made the conventional golf swing healthier due to the associated massive reduction of torsional forces when the FREE-RELEASE® Shoe is worn, which displaces the torsional forces harmful to the musculoskeletal system (quite comparable with the principle of the carving ski; the ski adopts or supports the rotation) in the so-called "hardware".

These improvements go far beyond other rather halfhearted attempts to address health problems arising in golf, by way of refined techniques.

From a scientific and medical point of view, the FREE-RELEASE-Method® can only be most warmly recommended to all medical colleagues active in sports medicine and interested in golf, but also to physiotherapists active in this field who are of course truly interested in the health of the golfers entrusted to their care.

In the interest of the health of all golfers (especially children and adolescents), I wish for a wide dissemination of this work, and I am convinced that the FREE-RELEASE-Method® will gain increasingly in acceptance.

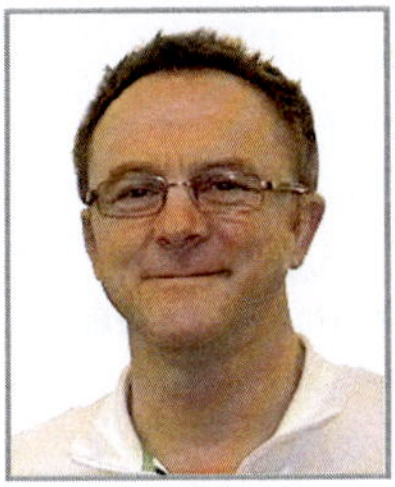

Dr. med.
Hans-Christoph Bosch
Stockach (Germany),
in July 2011

Greetings from Dr. med. Achim Rist

“After I looked closer at the overall system of “GAM FREE-RELEASE®”, I was able to successfully employ the method and the hardware with many of my golf patients. Based on interesting cases, I have published a case report and am convinced: Seen in terms of sports medicine and biomechanics, FREE-RELEASE® is the healthiest swing method and hardware for golfers worldwide!”

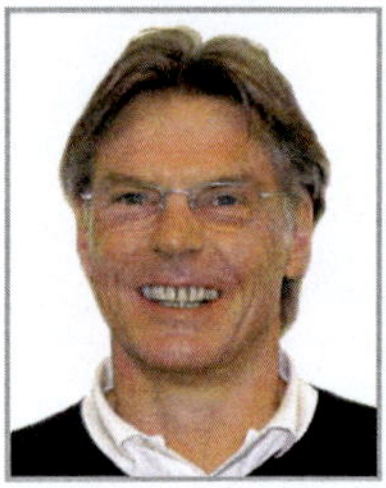

Dr. med. Achim Rist
Rennbahnklinik
Basel, Swiss
Olympic Medical Center

Letter of thanks from Jürgen Schuhmacher

Dear Mr. Drollinger,

Since I have been using the FREE-RELEASE® golf shoes for six months, I can confirm that this technique fully relieves my lower ankle joint. Due to a fracture in the left foot I have osteoarthritis in the ankle joint.

After a round of golf the joint pains were often so severe that at times I could hardly walk.

I even thought about quitting golf. Furthermore, I had great problems bringing the swing into a finish position.

Ever since I have been wearing your company's golf shoes I no longer have any complaints and my game of golf has become easier.

Jürgen Schuhmacher

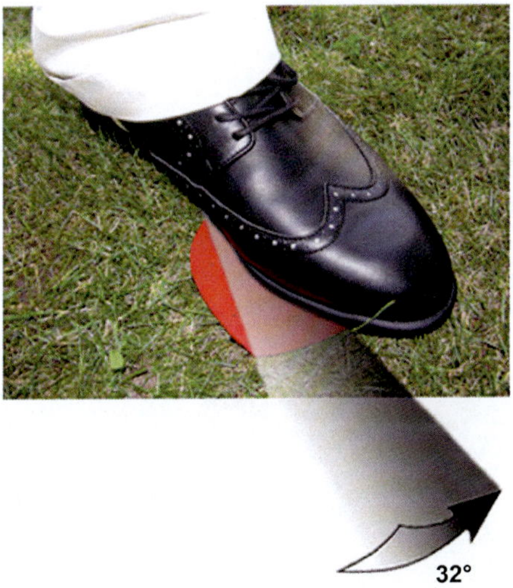

Greetings from Dietmar Hopp

Dear Mr. Drollinger,

...I have also implemented your suggestions for my swing with optimal success.

Result: handicap improvement from 12.7 to 8.6!

And there is still 'room' for improvement.

Best regards,
Dietmar Hopp

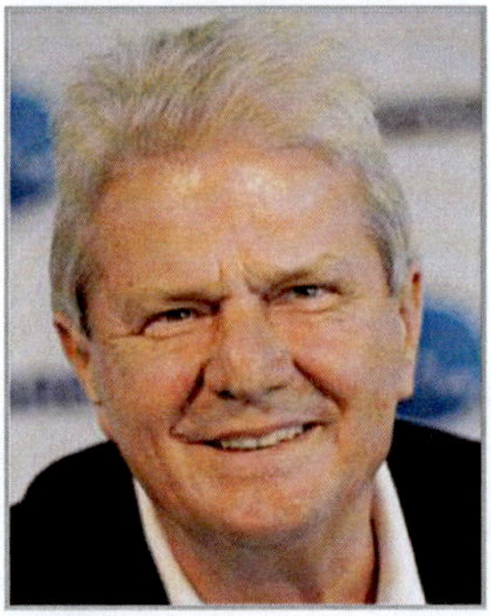

Dietmar Hopp
Founder of SAP

Greetings from Hamed Ibrahim

My name is Hamed, called "H". The Performance Pyramid, which has been developed by Frank Drollinger, includes the topic "Health Management" being one of the first priorities. In this connection, easing and relaxing, basically letting go, play a very significant role.

I am pleased to advice the developer of the FREE-RELEASE-Method® in such cases. For me, this shows that Frank thinks and acts "out of the box". Approximately 70% of my clients play golf. Most of them tell me that they have not yet reached their performance limit. This new approach can help everyone.

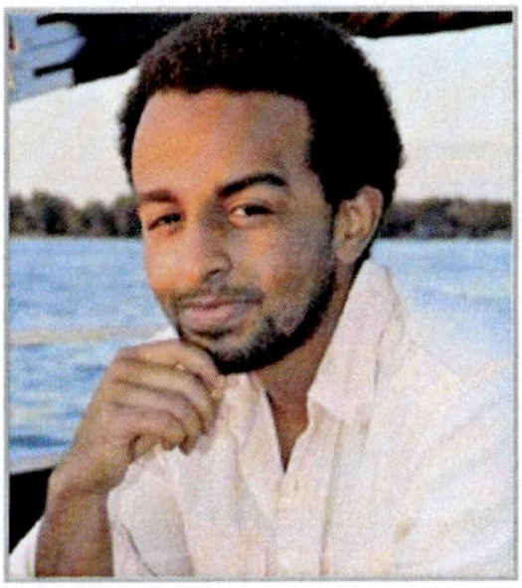

Hamed Ibrahim
Orlando, USA

Greetings from Cory McKim

"In addition to health protection for all golfers, the Golf-Active-Method FREE-RELEASE® particularly renders very great advantages for golf instructors:

We can tell a new, more efficient and healthier method story and consequently train millions of golfers, namely the 90% who no longer take lessons."

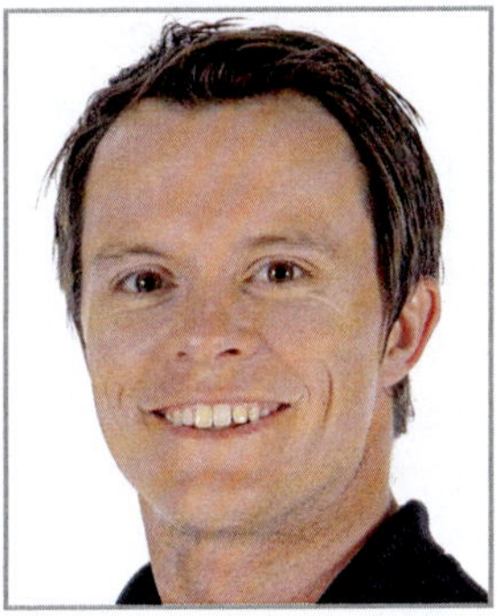

Cory McKim
PGA USA

Sports Medical Expert Dr. med. H.-J. Patzak on the issue „What will influence the world of golf"

In our daily work with athletes in both recreational sport and competitive sport, we repeatedly encounter the dilemma that sport causes health complaints and that treatment, even today's refined and intensive treatment, is no longer sufficient in order to enable an athlete to continue his or her hobby or profession. We are well aware that injuries in sports such as football and handball can lead to sports invalidity. Where golf is concerned, recreational golfers are generally unaware that injuries can lead to sports invalidity here as well.

Basically speaking, there are two aspects: Firstly, a competitive golfer who starts playing at a very early age, i.e. at pre-school age, can cause severe and lasting damage to his/her developing body due to constant repetitions involving significant strain placed on individual structures. Secondly, we have a rapidly growing number of recreational golfers who take up their hobby with existing injuries from other sports, who suffer complaints due to overuse or whose existing complaints force them to abandon their new hobby.

As sports medical experts we now have the possibility of drastically reducing the forces affecting the body after the moment of impact, based on the "FREE-RELEASE®" swing method developed by Frank Drollinger and the FREE-RELEASE® Shoe with a turnable sole, and to thus overcome the previously insurmountable problems in golf in combination with familiar treatments.

I have studied the FREE-RELEASE-Method® and the biomechanical background in detail and I am amazed at the precision with which strain can be defined and measured nowadays. I was surprised at the significant extent of strain where traditional swing techniques are in use with normal golf shoes, and at how drastically this strain can be reduced when the FREE-RELEASE-Method® and the FREE-

RELEASE® Shoe are used.

From the viewpoint of sports medicine, I am convinced that the FREE-RELEASE-Method® developed by Frank Drollinger will have a positive influence on golf worldwide.

Dr. med. H. – J. Patzak,
Sports Medical Expert

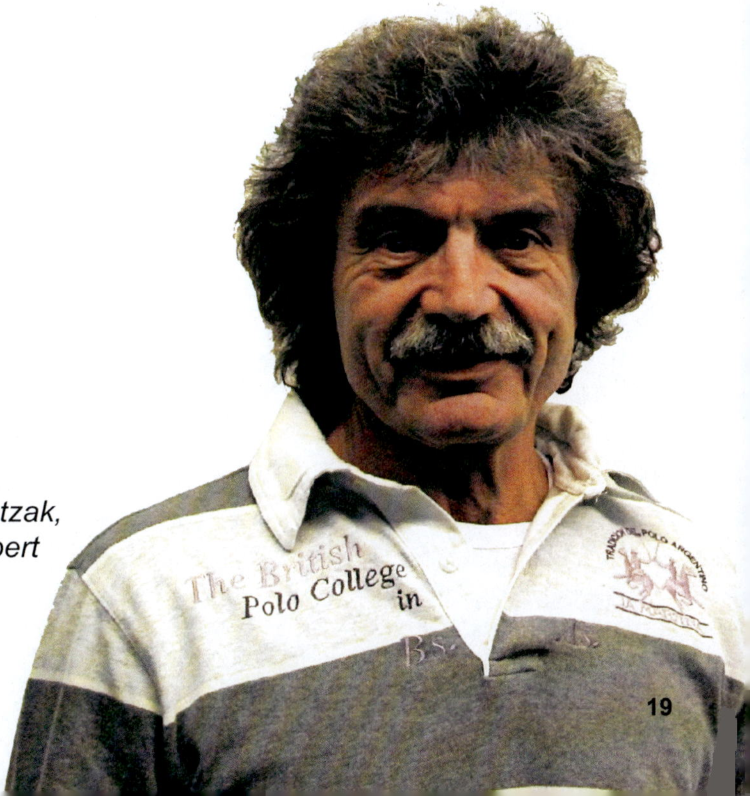

1. Golf-Biomechanic-Academy according to the FREE-RELEASE-Method® by Frank Drollinger

1.1. What is the Golf-Biomechanic-Academy?

We have made an international name for ourselves with the invention of the "Turning Shoe", the golf shoe with the turnable sole.

Since 2002 the idea of the patented "turning sole shoe" has expanded into an entire golf instruction and teaching method under the name "FREE-RELEASE®". In the meantime, international golf instructors as well as physicians and physiotherapists are being trained. The Golf-Biomechanic-Academy FREE-RELEASE® was established for this purpose in 2006.

We regularly train golf instructors, physiotherapists, orthopedists and sports medicine specialists according to the FREE-RELEASE-Method® in special advanced training courses there. The professional management of the training and advanced training sector is the responsibility of a national training team created specifically for this purpose. In addition to golf instructors, the team also includes sports scientists and biomechanists as well as an academically prestigious group of physicians.

In addition to the motional innovations of the FREE-RELEASE-Method®, our overall system also features the novelty aspect that the golf instructor no longer has the sole say about the various concerns of golfers and athletes.

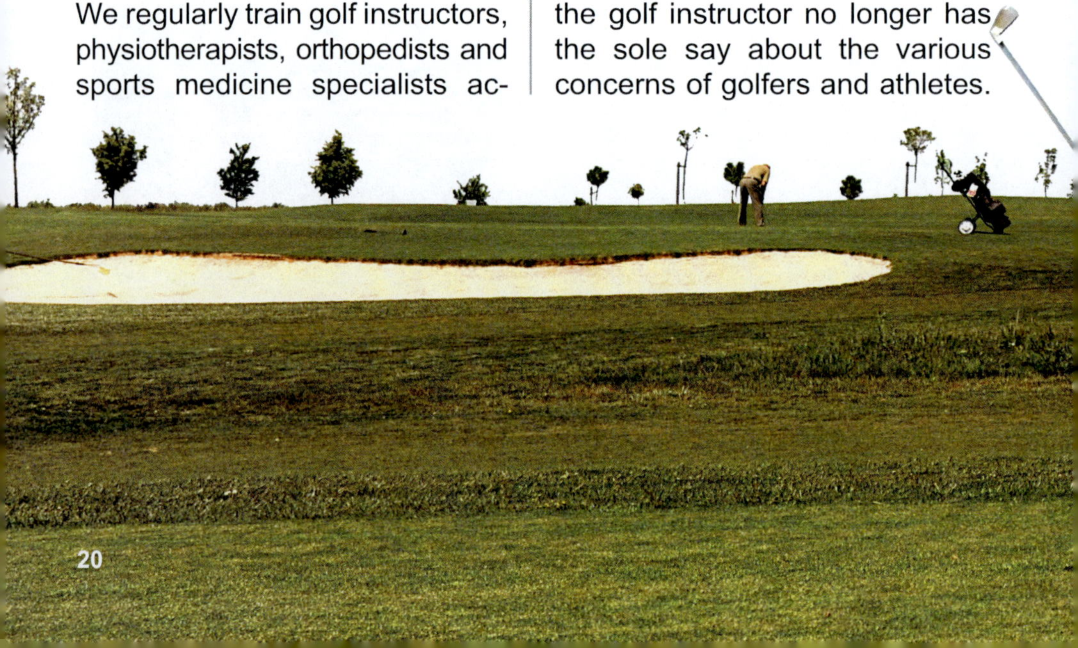

The golf instructor is in fact part of an expert system. The golf instructor in our system does not work single-handedly, but is in a team integrated into a network comprised of specially trained experts in the following fields:

- GOLF-MEDICAL-COACH
- GOLF-PHYSIO-COACH (MED)
- GOLF-ORTHO-COACH
- GOLF-PERSONAL-COACH
- GOLF-ATHLETIC-TRAINER
- GOLF-MED-DENT-COACH
- GOLF-MENTAL-COACH
- GOLF-OPTIC-EXPERT
- GOLF-NUTRITION-EXPERT
- GOLF-BIOMECHANIC-PRO (MED)

As a result, "Safety First" – the first and foremost concept in health and injury protection – is implemented for the athletes, and at the same time an optimal development of the performance of individual athletes is enabled. The golf instructors trained by us as "GOLF-BIOMECHANIC-PRO" play an essential role in this respect as network members. This is a system that is long since well-known and successfully practiced in other sports.

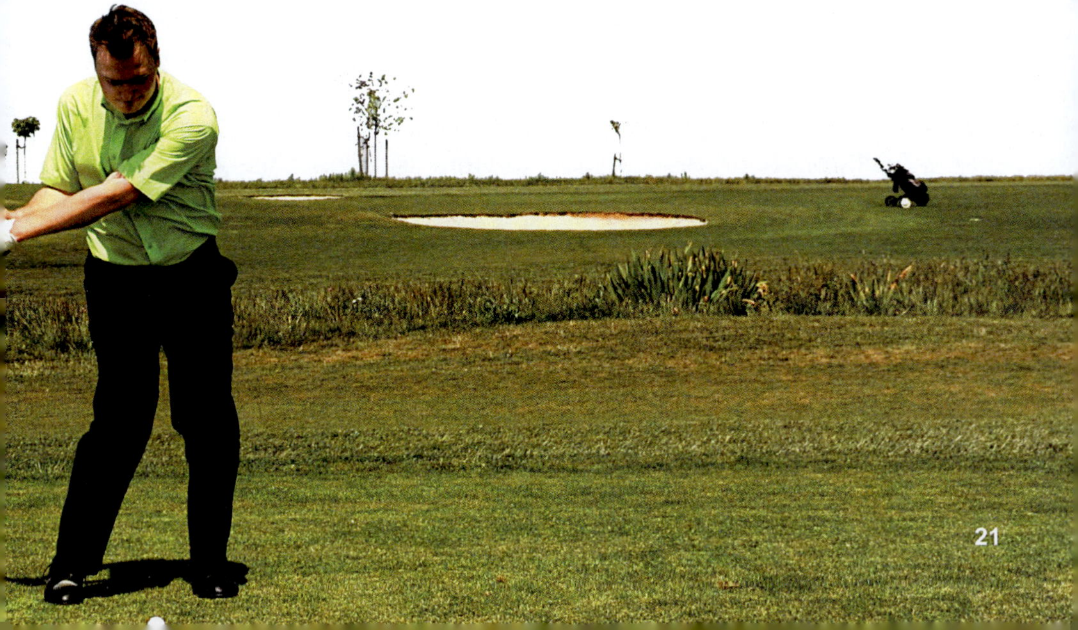

1.1.a. Seminars at the Golf-Biomechanic-Academy according to the FREE-RELEASE-Method®

In addition to courses for coaches, golf instructors and association decision-makers we also offer seminars for our highly appreciated end customers at the Golf-Biomechanic-Academy FREE-RELEASE®. It was always a thorn in my side that high-end offers were frequently reserved for high-performance sports.

We are attached to the entire community of golfers. That is why there is no reason for us to keep amateur golfers away from our Golf-Biomechanic-Academy.

From my point of view, most amateur golfers – regardless of handicap – also achieve peak performances measured against their circumstances.

Amateur golfers are additionally burdened through profession or household circumstances. In contrast, a pro golfer trains about 10 hours a day. That is why we should not underestimate the performances of amateur players, but respect them to the highest degree.

Based on representative surveys it is known that over 90% of the members in German golf clubs no longer take lessons with a golf instructor. If you deduct the number of those who have sponsored training because they are members of a team or the like, the real rate of instruction or training is even worse.

In this case we also encounter a phenomenon that is often referred to as “emotional intelligence”. Without reflecting on this phenomenon in more detail, club members know exactly why they no longer take lessons with an instructor for conventional golf swing method:

It does not bring golfers a step further!

Learning progress for many golfers is apparently exhausted with conventional method.

50% of this inactive group of instruction-resistant golfers would renounce their attitude and resume golf instruction if they were certain of their success. This certainty of success can be conveyed with a guarantee of improvement.

Learning only makes sense as long as tangible progress ensues.

For this purpose we calculate your performance data at the start and end of further training with lasers, Doppler radar, high-speed cameras (60 images/second), and balance measurements.

We know from experience that you will improve with our new swing method.

My assistant will gladly answer all of your questions about our seminar series at:

education@free-release.com

We also gladly offer additional individual or group courses (medical groups, teams) above and beyond our regular program. The educational and training framework is tailored to your schedule and technical requirements.

Your best golf game lies in the future! Best wishes,

Frank Drollinger
www.golf-active-method.com
www.golf-biomechanic-pro.com

GOLF-BIOMECHANIC-ACADEMY.COM
Golf-Health & biomechanical, neurological & kinematical Swing-Programming for Performance Improvement according to the FREE - RELEASE - Method® by Frank Drollinger

1.2. Golf – a sport with risks

1.2.a. Injury protection & performance improvement

The list of players absent from the Tour due to injury is long. At the same time, golf pros try to improve their performance by all means in order to remain competitive.

Immediately after the fundamentals of injury & health protection, the Golf-Biomechanic-Academy concentrates on improving the golfer's individual performance.

Performance improvements are solely the result of an optimization and simplification of conventional golf swing biomechanics. On average, we achieve an improvement of about 15% among pros and 25% among amateurs in this connection.

The performance improvements achieved in this connection can be demonstrated specifically in the Smash 7 values by means of measurements.

In an interview from January 2011, Sandra Gal explained that she only reached 30% of her performance capability. As a top athlete, she perceived with her emotional intelligence that beyond her previous swinging instruction there is still a way to achieve more performance capability than in the past.

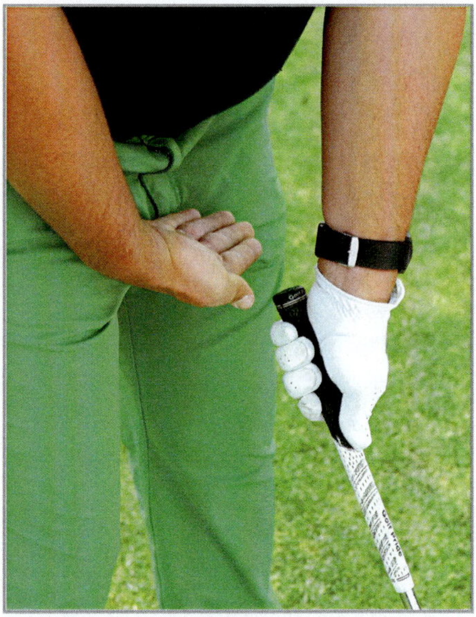

Surely not a performance improvement by 70%, but certainly by 20%!

In fact, a 10% performance improvement would already be enough for Sandra to advance into the elite group of Top 10 players. On the other hand, if she continues as previously, such a place in the ranking list is merely a stroke of luck. Above all, adherence to previous achievements would be highly unprofessional, since a pro has to take advantage of all permissible options in order to be competitive.

The key to being successful in pro golf competition lies in the functional golf biomechanics developed by us.

This involves avoiding injuries and physical complaints that are typical and widespread in the golf world, by means of a physiological golf swing motion.

Furthermore, our progressive biomechanics enables an enhanced transfer of energy to the golf ball, measurably improved target precision of ball flight, and a repeatability of this "high-end" quality.

"Rory McIlroy, the player ranked number one in the current world ranking in May 2012, hits 50% of fairways with 100 tee shots. He could improve his performance by a maximum of 100%, but only if he switches to the movement principles of the FREE-RELEASE-Method®."

Frank Drollinger

1.2.b. FREE-RELEASE®-Strategy for performance improvement among golfers

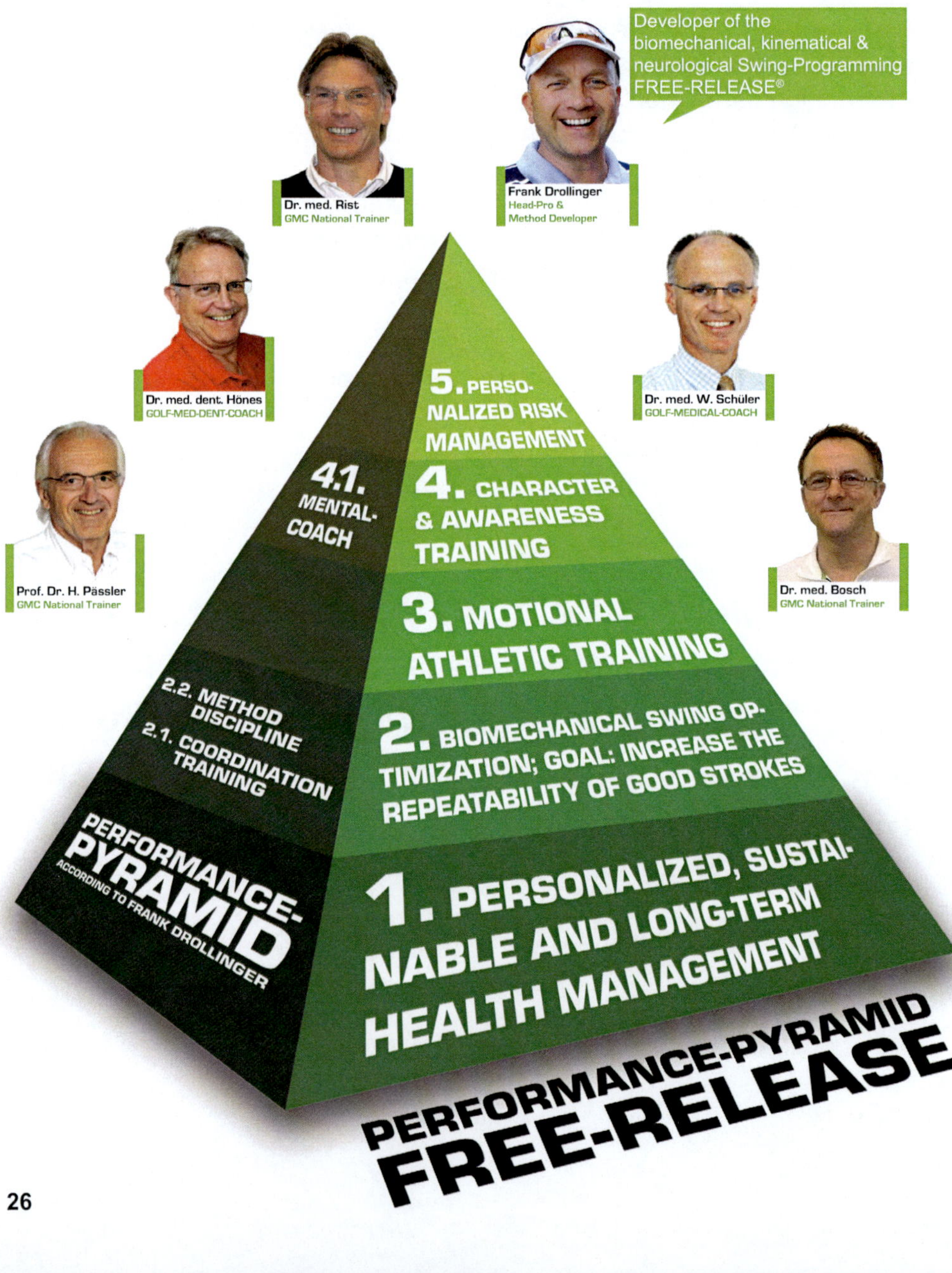
Developer of the biomechanical, kinematical & neurological Swing-Programming FREE-RELEASE®
Dr. med. Rist
GMC National Trainer
Frank Drollinger
Head-Pro & Method Developer
Dr. med. dent. Hönes
GOLF-MED-DENT-COACH
Dr. med. W. Schüler
GOLF-MEDICAL-COACH
Prof. Dr. H. Pässler
GMC National Trainer
Dr. med. Bosch
GMC National Trainer
5. PERSONALIZED RISK MANAGEMENT
4.1. MENTAL-COACH
4. CHARACTER & AWARENESS TRAINING
3. MOTIONAL ATHLETIC TRAINING
2.2. METHOD DISCIPLINE
2.1. COORDINATION TRAINING
2. BIOMECHANICAL SWING OPTIMIZATION; GOAL: INCREASE THE REPEATABILITY OF GOOD STROKES
PERFORMANCE-PYRAMID
ACCORDING TO FRANK DROLLINGER
1. PERSONALIZED, SUSTAINABLE AND LONG-TERM HEALTH MANAGEMENT
PERFORMANCE-PYRAMID
FREE-RELEASE

”The Turning Shoe is two shoes in one. Up until ball impact it is a very normal golf shoe, and after the ball impact it becomes a sports medical product which protects the golfer against the unhealthy influence of forces.”

Frank Drollinger

Basis of the Performance-Pyramid according to the FREE-RELEASE-Methode® by Frank Drollinger

Sector: Health Management

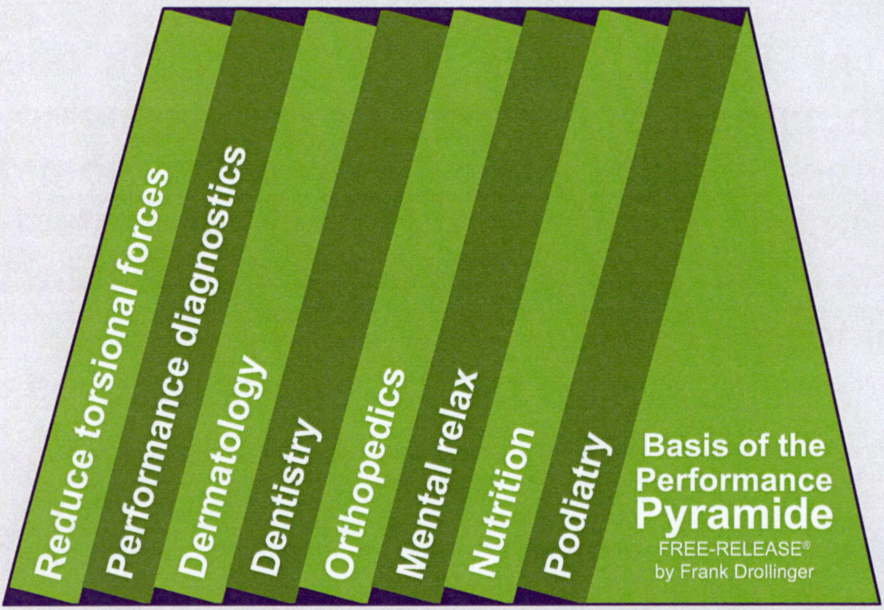
Reduce torsional forces
Performance diagnostics
Dermatology
Dentistry
Orthopedics
Mental relax
Nutrition
Podiatry
Basis of the Performance Pyramide
FREE-RELEASE®
by Frank Drollinger

“As long as hundreds of scientists and medical experts commit to the same principles of sports science, namely to ‘do everything in order to minimize the risk of injury for golfers/athletes’ and to ‘improve their health,’ I am in the best company and fighting for the right cause.
The International Olympic Sports Federation has also anchored these fundamental ethical regulations in its articles.
I cannot and will not accept that individual functionaries within the German Olympic Sports Confederation, within the German Golf Association (DGV), the USGA, IGF and R&A actively work against these principles by failing to fulfill their obligations, by failing to transfer the issue while being fully aware of the consequences in sports medicine, or who deliberately and actively prevent the introduction of health management, for this definitely attitude does not reflect the social and intellectual competence of golfers.”

Frank Drollinger, June 2012

1.2.c. The 5-Easy-Upgrades

1. Set-Up:

Axis parallelism of the feet, knees, pelvis (Fig. 1), shoulders, head, chin high (Fig. 2), hand's width distance (Fig. 3 + 4), and stance width so that the right leg can accelerate the pelvis parallel to the target horizon (Fig. 5).

Upper body-pelvic angle is approx. 40 degrees (see page 80). Establish vertical and horizontal balance.

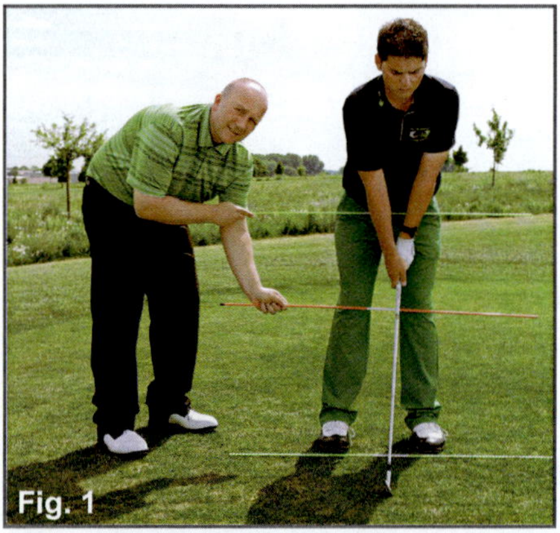
Fig. 1

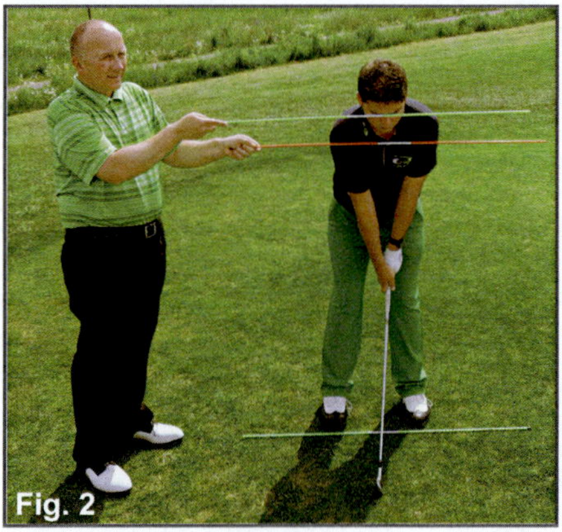
Fig. 2

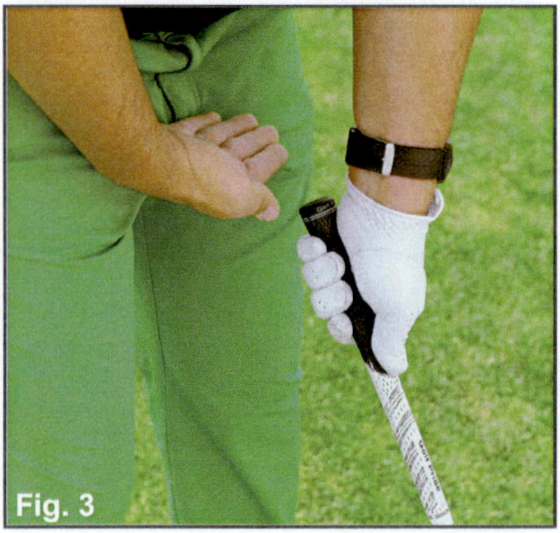
Fig. 3

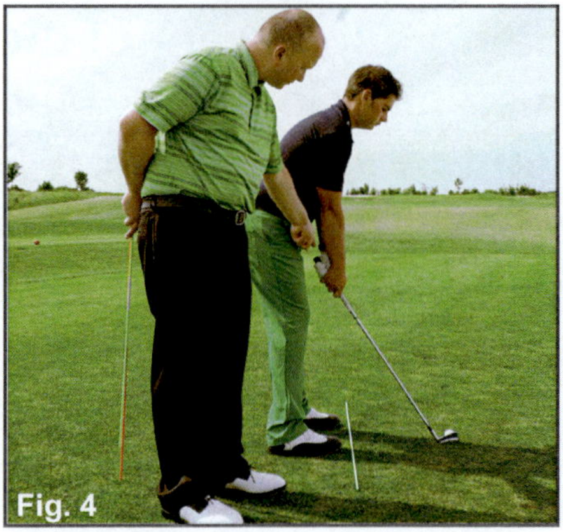
Fig. 4

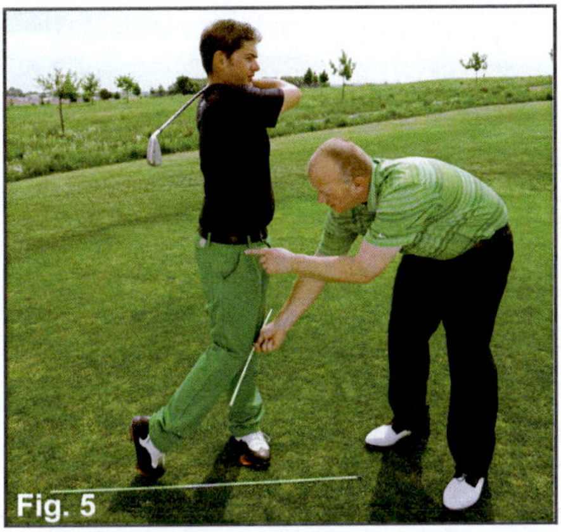

Fig. 5

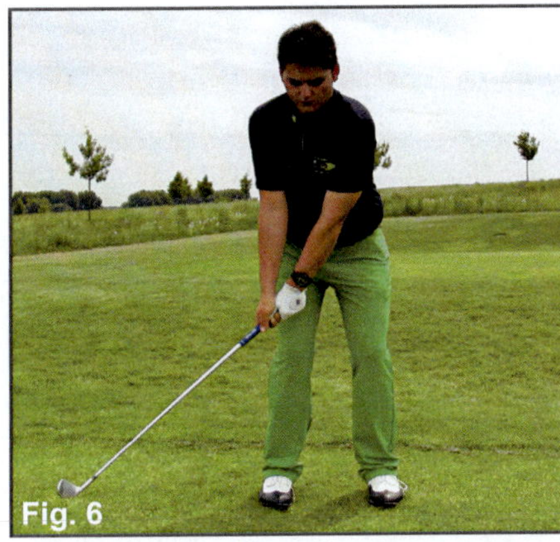

Fig. 6

2. Backswing:

Release right hip and shoulder as well as back of the left hand; as a synchronous “Y”, this pushes the arms and the club towards the right thigh without bending (Fig. 6); from here (increase the angle in your wrists vertically by hinging them upright) angle the hand. The left upper arm remains close to the upper body. Movement occurs backwards and upwards. The left arm remains stretched; the pelvis turns up to 45 degrees and shoulder up to 90 degrees (Fig. 7).

The shaft intersects the right shoulder. The swing plane is parallel to the setup position; slow motional execution is important in order to keep the body's center of gravity fixed and to maintain balance throughout the entire backswing phase. (Fig. 10 + 12)

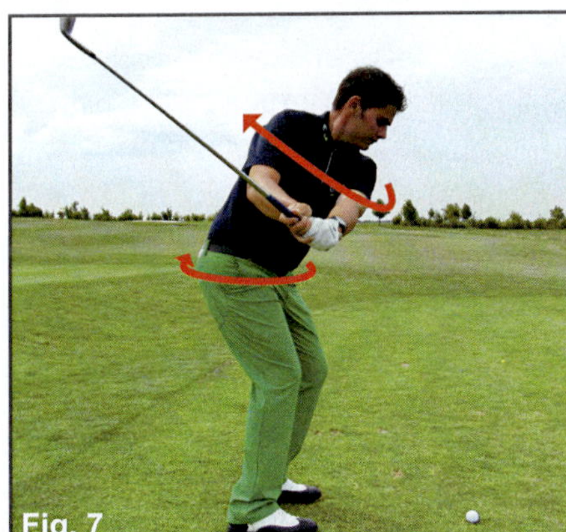

Fig. 7

See page 85 for the end position of the backswing

3. Downswing:

The downswing starts with an active, controlled rotational impulse in the big toe of the right foot (Fig. 8), the aim being to use the large muscles of the right leg together with the gluteal muscles on the right side in order to accelerate the pelvis into X-factor-2 (ball impact) and then into X-factor-3 (finish position).

Until the moment of ball impact the pelvis moves 67.5 degrees in the FREE-RELEASE-Method®.

Active legwork implemented through the dynamics of the rotational impulse enables a significant improvement in driving accuracy and GIR due to the generation of up to 10 times more energy in comparison to acceleration using the diagonal abdominal muscles alone (Rory McIlroy, ESPN, Sport Science Video).

Ideal acceleration of the hips using diagonal abdominal muscles at the rate of 25% and 75% due to active legwork. Rory McIlroy* and Sergio Gargia* could achieve a 100% improvement in this respect.

*(DA 50%; as at April 2012, europeantour.com, STAT)

In addition, sudden twisting using the diagonal abdominal muscles alone in order to accelerate the hips into the moment of ball impact is not controllable or physiologically beneficial. Injuries to the lumbar region and the hips can be expected. This uncontrolled acceleration of the hips also has an extremely negative impact on the progress of the body's center of gravity (three-dimensional, diagonal "8" traced).

Active legwork is compensated by the faster arm movement; ideally the two rotations will converge at the moment of ball impact; the left wrist is triggered by rotational forces and accelerates the club head shortly before the moment of impact; there is a shift in weight shortly before the moment of impact. (Fig. 9)

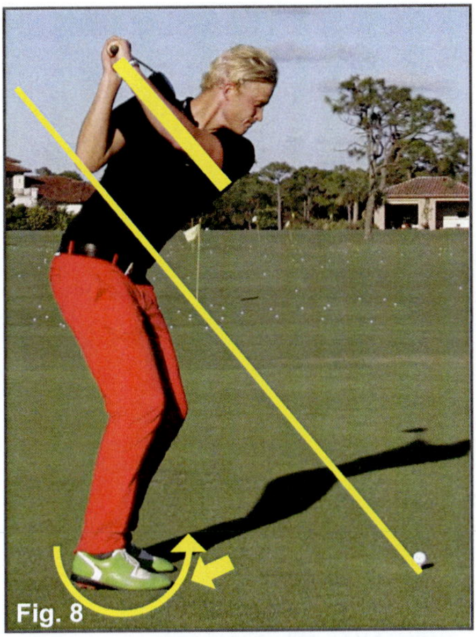
Fig. 8

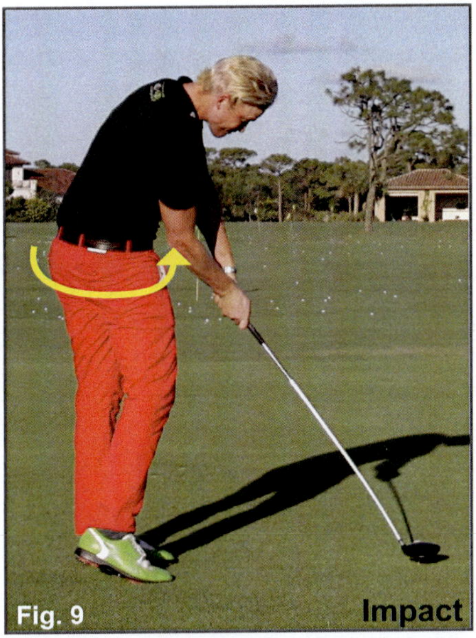
Fig. 9
Impact

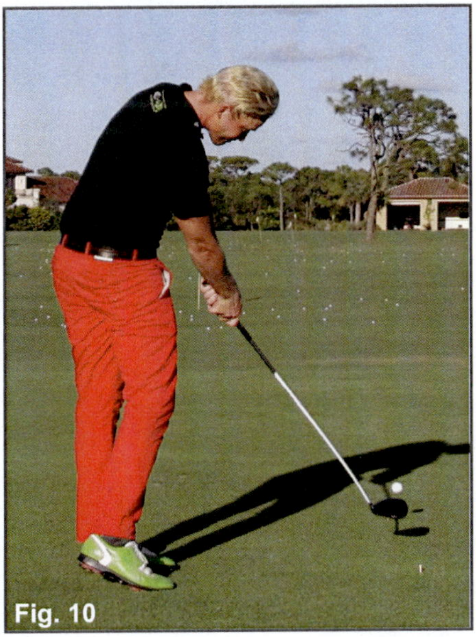
Fig. 10

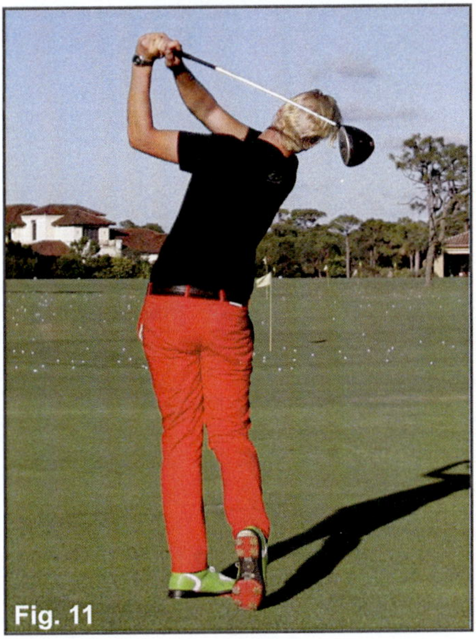
Fig. 11

4. Ball impact:

Ball impact ideally occurs with a 90 degree angle of club face and ball; tolerance in this connection is plus/minus 2.5 degrees (Fig. 9); pelvis and shoulder turn further; if the Turning Shoe is used, the Turning Shoe releases after ball impact, and from here reduces the torsional forces arising (Fig. 10).

5. Finish:

Pelvis and shoulder are ideally at a 90 degree angle; club is placed on the left shoulder; this position is held for approx. four seconds; eyes follow the ball flight until landing and the rollout (Fig. 11).

”The Turning Shoe is the most ingenious invention in golf sport. Its health benefits can be compared with the success story of the helmet in alpine skiing. Upon careful consideration the Turning Shoe is the only way to comply with modern regulations of the United Nations, to improve the social progress and life quality of people, of the Olympic movement, to make every effort to reduce the risk of injury for athletes, the WADA Charter, to improve athletes’ health, of the Rules of Golf, to protect one’s competitors and oneself against injury, and contractual obligations not to expose members, pupils and customers to health risks.”

Frank Drollinger

1.2.d. „Safety First“ with pros and amateurs

The Rules of Golf and the IOC Charter require that protection of the athlete's health be given the highest priority by all players in professional as well as amateur golf.

With that said, "Safety First" for athletes is also the guiding principle in golf, because golf has been an Olympic sport since 2009, and all organizations have undertaken in writing to observe the IOC Charter.

It is frequently underestimated quite how significant the task of improved health protection is, particularly in golf.

That is why we have prepared an extract from the database on injuries among professional golfers which shows that practically every Tour player has suffered from serious orthopedic complaints and/or severe injuries to the musculoskeletal system.

For instance, not only Tom Watson and Jesper Parnevik already had hip endoprostheses implanted at a relatively young age, but many other pros have also under-gone significant operative interventions.

Millions of dedicated hobby golfers face the same fate as their professional colleagues.

Injuries and complaints of the musculoskeletal system as a result of non-physiological motion of the conventional swing model are also common among amateur golfers. This shows that the anatomy of our musculoskeletal system – the ligaments, bones, intervertebral discs and articular cartilage – were not created for the golf swing according to the sequence of movements described by Ben Hogan.

Prof. Dr. Bergmann from the Charité Medical Center in Berlin has determined through corresponding measurements that a temperature increase of up to 43 degrees Celsius takes place in artificial hip joints after one hour of "walking", i.e. a sequence of movements without torsion affecting joints.

Due to these findings, my research partners and I have come to the conclusion that the temperature increases in a joint structure will be even greater if – as with the conventional swing motion – additional torsional and shearing forces as well as vibrations affect the joint or if increased joint friction occurs.

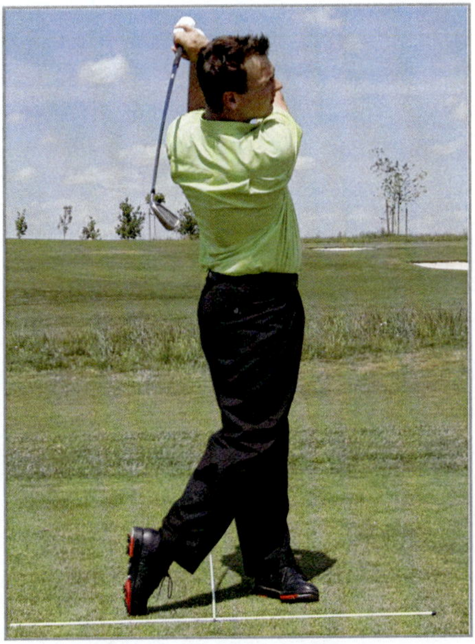

Stress-free finish position
Alexander Groschopp
FREE-RELEASE® National Trainer
One of the best students of Frank Drollinger

Thermal damage to joints after a few minutes of training on the driving range is therefore unavoidable with the previous swing motion.

The treacherous thing about such micro-injuries – which frequently occur on the articular cartilage of the knee, for instance – lies in the fact that the cartilage does not have any nerves which signal pain or injuries. Pains cease only once the cartilage structure is almost completely destroyed and thereby irreparably damaged.

Hence cartilage protection and joint prophylaxis have to be deliberately and specifically pursued at a point in time in which no joint complaints are present.

This especially applies to children and adolescents during the growth phase.

The golf swing according to the passive method developed by Ben Hogan generates violent stress impacts of more than 14 newton meters (Nm) per kg of body weight on the golfer's joint structures – where the "textbook correct" swing is executed.

If the swing is executed incorrectly, for instance in compensatory false postures, the peak load values continue to increase. We have ascertained these and other measurement data in scientific examinations with prestigious research institutions of various universities.

Our Golf-Active-Method FREE-RELEASE® reduces the measured loads by nearly 100%. Particularly

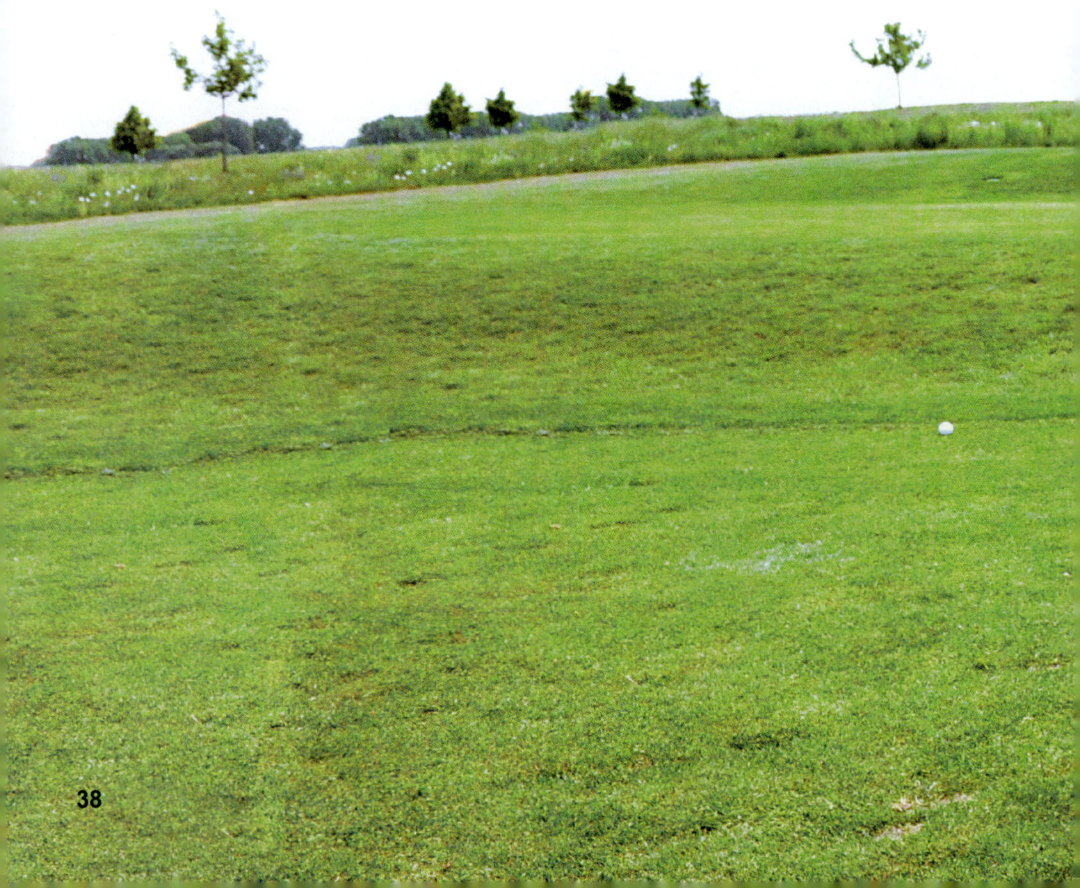

for physicians and holistic medical practitioners, our system enables symptoms of complaints and pain to be treated on the biomechanical causative level.

Primary, secondary and tertiary prevention should prevent health impairments, but also help protect athletes who already have injuries against recurring injuries.

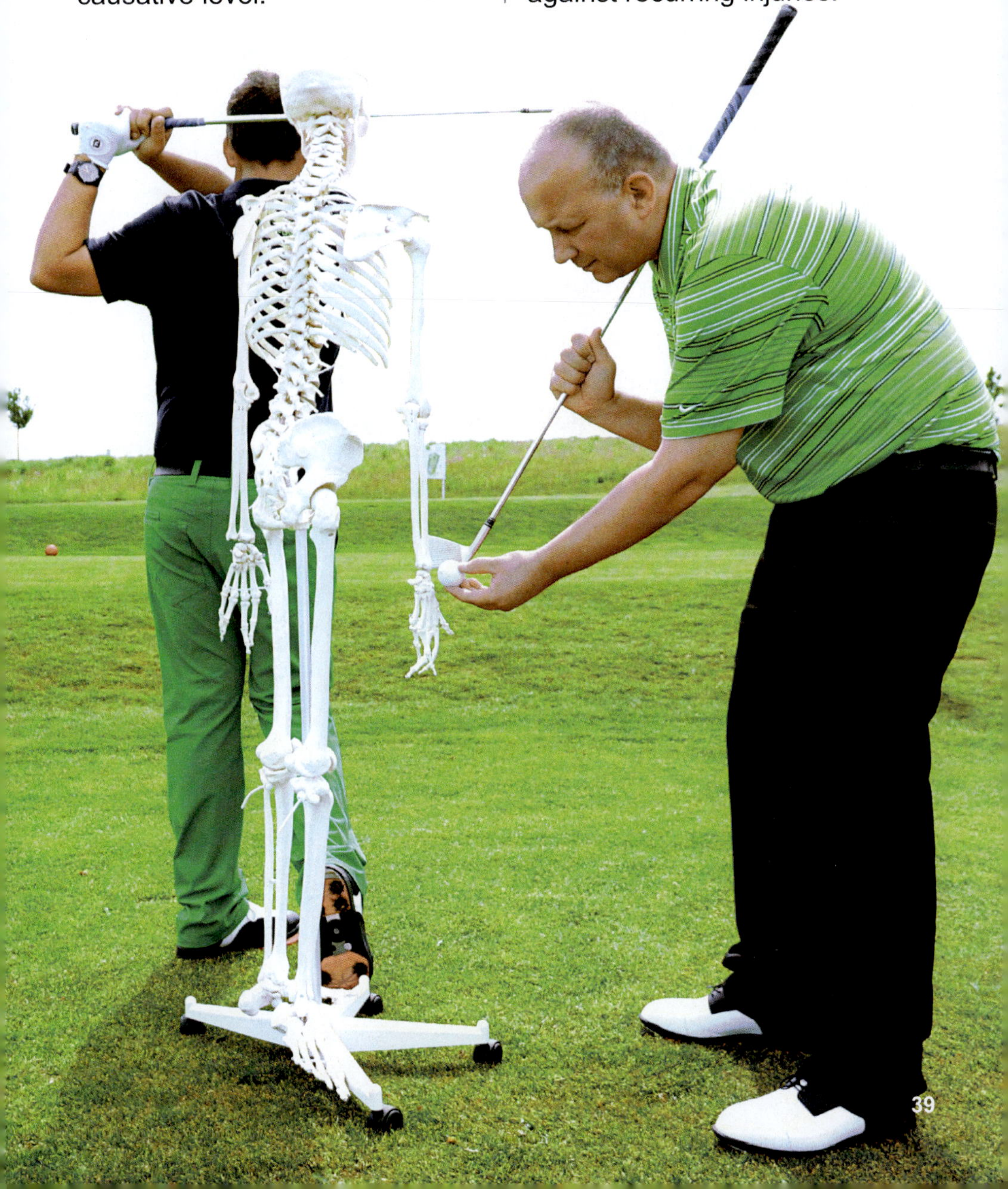

1.2.e. Playing golf when in pain

If hopeful talents fight against the dysfunctional biomechanics of the conventional golf swing and are therefore already written off in sports coverage, we perceive such situations as a genuine challenge to prove that such players in particular can obtain the proverbial polish of a "raw diamond" through the biomechanics of our swing method. Erstwhile losers become European Tour players.

Parents, coaches, youth coordinators and club executive boards should keep this in mind.

Our research efforts have revealed that injuries – as they have become known to a broad public in the case of Tiger Woods – are by no means an isolated case.

It is not the end of the world if an athletic career grinds to a halt. But an athletic career – in the truest sense of the word – should not come to an end because of an avoidable injury. That is why injury protection is a fundamental prerequisite for sustainable career development. Professional athletes do not talk willingly about injuries because it could scare away potential sponsors. This is a thoroughly understandable calculation that once again shows that our society stigmatizes physical weaknesses or infirmities and thus indirectly promotes the consumption of painkillers.

However, the use of painkillers that is particularly widespread in golf is to be condemned in terms of sporting ethics. After all, it ultimately brings about a performance improvement through the administration of medication. Consequently, the consumption of painkillers is and will be classified by experts as doping.

Solely for this reason every golf athlete should confront the considerable risk of injury by taking advantage of our system. I originally developed the hardware and software of our swing system only for personal therapy. My pains and injuries have been eliminated since that time.

Dr. Achim Rist from the Rennbahnklinik Basel (Swiss Olympic Medical Center), who is the leader of our group of physicians in the FREE-RELEASE® training team, also determined within the course of his patient study that a pain-free game of golf is made possible through our hardware system for patients with orthopedic complaints typical of golf.

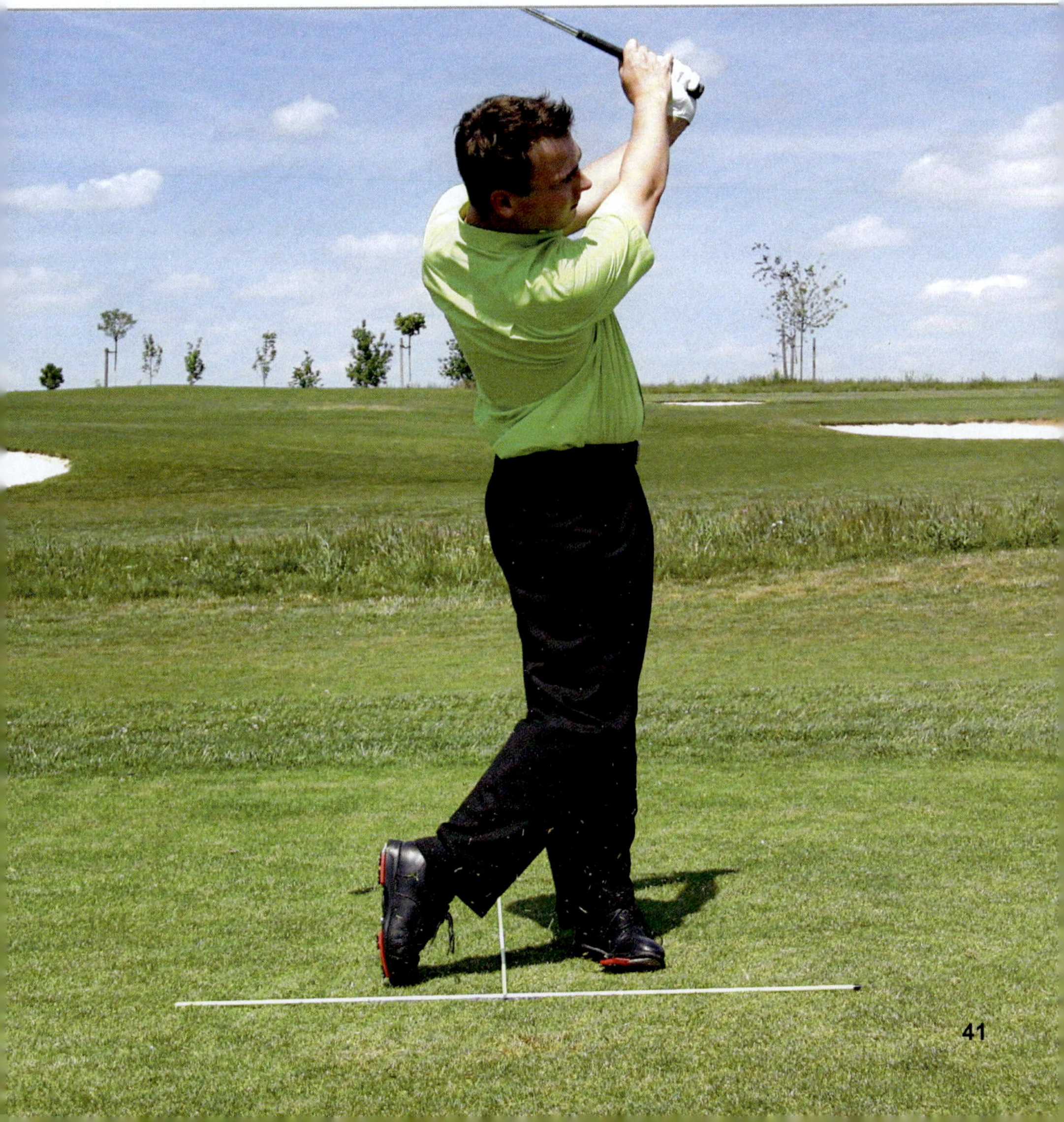

1.2.f. Health protection for children

Children are particularly vulnerable to injury during the growth phase.

Hardly any attention is paid to the protection of articular cartilage among children, although the cartilage structures will be massively impaired through the previous golf swing. Because cartilage can no longer regenerate, parents, golf instructors, youth coaches, and youth coordinators must handle this situation very responsibly.

The Golf-Active-Method FREE-RELEASE® is the world's only

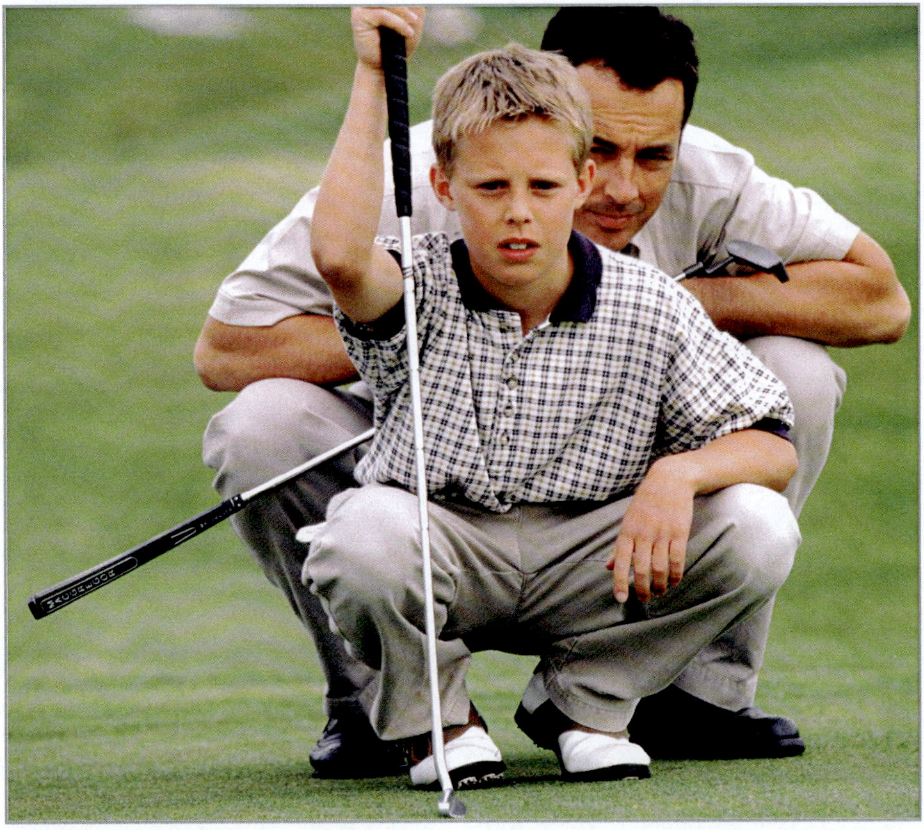

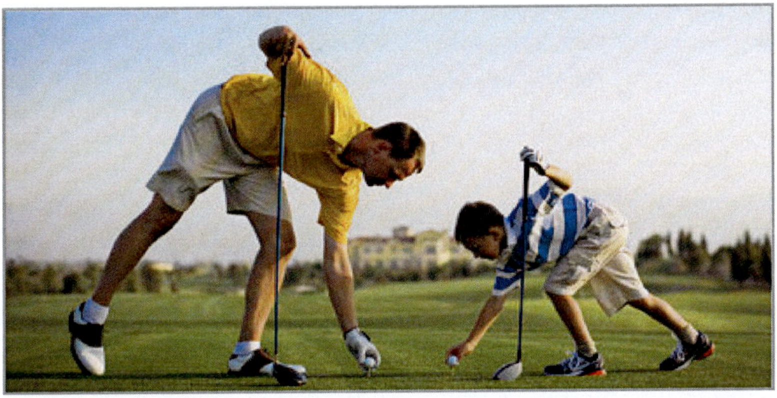

functional option along this route. When I observe responsible parents who are concerned about the health of their children, then I notice that the vast majority of them do a great deal in order to protect their children.

For instance, it has become quite normal that children wear helmets for passive injury and health protection when skiing. Parents are still lacking this future-oriented approach when it comes to golf. Therefore we must do everything necessary to sensitize parents to the fact that the enormous stress influences of the golf swing can lead to serious long-term orthopedic impairments, particularly among children and adolescents.

At the same time, parents must know that active protection against these dangers is possible.

Our system, with which the stress influences on the musculoskeletal system can be substantially reduced, ranks foremost in this connection.

This means that children will be actively protected against influence of forces through torsion, shearing forces, friction and vibration.

Olympic Sports	Active Health Protection	Passive Health Protection	Olympic Protective Regulations
Bobsled		x	Helmet
Boxing	x	x	Helmet, gloves, mouth guard, groin protector
Fencing	x		Jacket, breeches, helmet (with mask), gloves, plastron
Football (soccer)		x	Shin guard
Hockey (field hockey)		x	Shin guard, mouth guard
Ice hockey		x	Helmet, knee & arm protectors, neck guard, gloves, mouth guard, shoulder pads, body
Judo		x	Mouth guard, groin protector
Kayak		x	Helmet, life preserver
Golf			
Cycling (mountain bike)		x	Helmet, gloves
Cycling (road race)		x	Helmet
Equestrianism (jumping)		x	Helmet, protective vest
Equestrianism (eventing)		x	Helmet
Rugby		x	Mouth guard
Taekwondo	x	x	Protective vest, groin protector, shin guard, helmet
Triathlon (bicycle)		x	Helmet
Alpine skiing		x	Helmet
Ski jumping		x	Helmet
Freestyle skiing		x	Helmet
Snowboarding		x	Helmet
Water polo		x	Water polo cap with ear protection

Mandatory in Competition / Tournament	Mandatory in Recreational Sports	Voluntary Protection
Helmet		
Helmet, gloves, mouth guard, groin protector	Helmet, gloves, mouth guard, groin protector	
Jacket, breeches, helmet (with mask), gloves, plastron	Jacket, breeches, helmet (with mask), gloves	
Shin guard		Shin guard
Shin guard, mouth guard		
Helmet, knee & arm protectors, neck guard, gloves, mouth guard, shoulder pads, body	Helmet, knee & arm protectors, neck guard, gloves, mouth guard, shoulder pads, body	
Mouth guard, groin protector		Groin protector
Helmet, life preserver	Helmet, life preserver	
Helmet, gloves		
Helmet		Gloves
Helmet, protective vest	Helmet	
Helmet	Helmet	
Mouth guard	Mouth guard	Groin protector
Protective vest, groin protector, shin guard, helmet	Protective vest, groin protector	
Helmet	Helmet	
Helmet		(Varies by country)
Helmet		
Helmet		
Helmet		Back protector
Water polo cap with ear protection	Water polo cap with ear protection	

2. Turning Shoe Health Promoter

The Turning Shoe Health Promoter is a pure sports medical product which provides active health protection for golfers and golfing children during a single golf swing.

a test of golf shoes from various brands with conventional shoe sole systems it was determined that due to their technical design and static, fixed sole systems of all brands have significant and

Comparative test of golf shoes: 2005/2010

		Protection against		
Provider	**Ø price in $**	**Torsions**	**Supinations**	**Shearing force**
Adi	200	Poor (6.0)	Poor (6.0)	Poor (6.0)
Nik	220	Poor (6.0)	Poor (6.0)	Poor (6.0)
Fo	180	Poor (6.0)	Poor (6.0)	Poor (6.0)
Ec	210	Poor (6.0)	Poor (6.0)	Poor (6.0)
Pu	160	Poor (6.0)	Poor (6.0)	Poor (6.0)
Ge	200	Poor (6.0)	Poor (6.0)	Poor (6.0)
Du	140	Poor (6.0)	Poor (6.0)	Poor (6.0)
United Golfers	**319**	**Very good (1.2)**	**Very good (1.0)**	**Very good (1.4)**
Cal	180	Poor (6.0)	Poor (6.0)	Poor (6.0)
Bit	110	Poor (6.0)	Poor (6.0)	Poor (6.0)
Oal	210	Poor (6.0)	Poor (6.0)	Poor (6.0)

In contrast to a protective helmet (e.g. in racing), reducing the risk of injury is not passive, but active.

It has an intelligent turning shoe sole which only functions **after** ball impact due to torsional forces. In

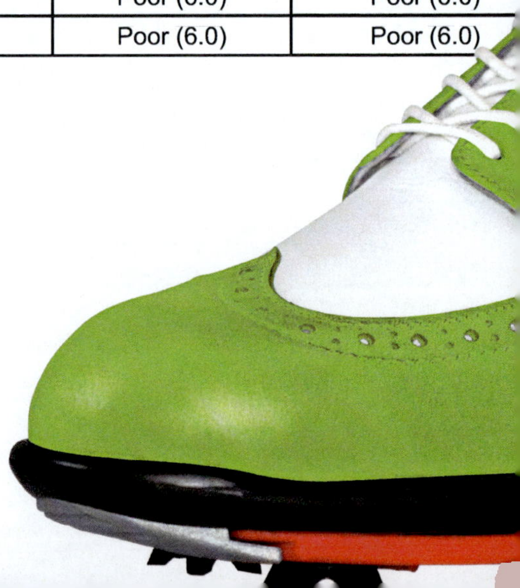

harmful effects on the golfer. Only the Turning Shoe Health Promoter was able to reduce loads by up to 99% after ball impact due to the turning shoe sole.

Protection against			
Joint friction	**Anatomical structures limiting impairment**	**Fragile impairment structures among children**	**Spinal torsions**
Poor (6.0)	Poor (6.0)	Poor (6.0)	Poor (6.0)
Poor (6.0)	Poor (6.0)	Poor (6.0)	Poor (6.0)
Poor (6.0)	Poor (6.0)	Poor (6.0)	Poor (6.0)
Poor (6.0)	Poor (6.0)	Poor (6.0)	Poor (6.0)
Poor (6.0)	Poor (6.0)	Poor (6.0)	Poor (6.0)
Poor (6.0)	Poor (6.0)	Poor (6.0)	Poor (6.0)
Poor (6.0)	Poor (6.0)	Poor (6.0)	Poor (6.0)
ery good (1.4)	**Very good (1.4)**	**Very good (1.0)**	**Very good (1.0)**
Poor (6.0)	Poor (6.0)	Poor (6.0)	Poor (6.0)
Poor (6.0)	Poor (6.0)	Poor (6.0)	Poor (6.0)
6.0)	6.0)	Poor (6.0)	Poor (6.0)

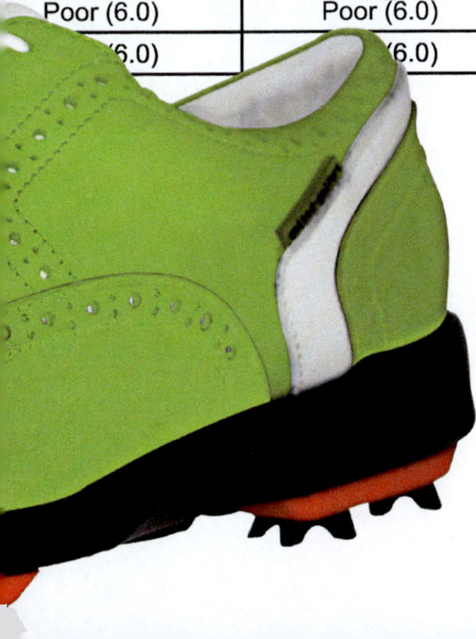

Turning Shoe Health Promoter

If the body rotation is supposed to happen in a physiological manner, i.e. without the harmful effect of shearing, torsional and frictional forces, vibration, intervertebral disc pressure and injury to articular cartilage, ligaments, tendons and intervertebral discs, this can only be achieved by means of the Turning Shoe, which prevents unnatural torsion of the musculoskeletal system after ball impact.

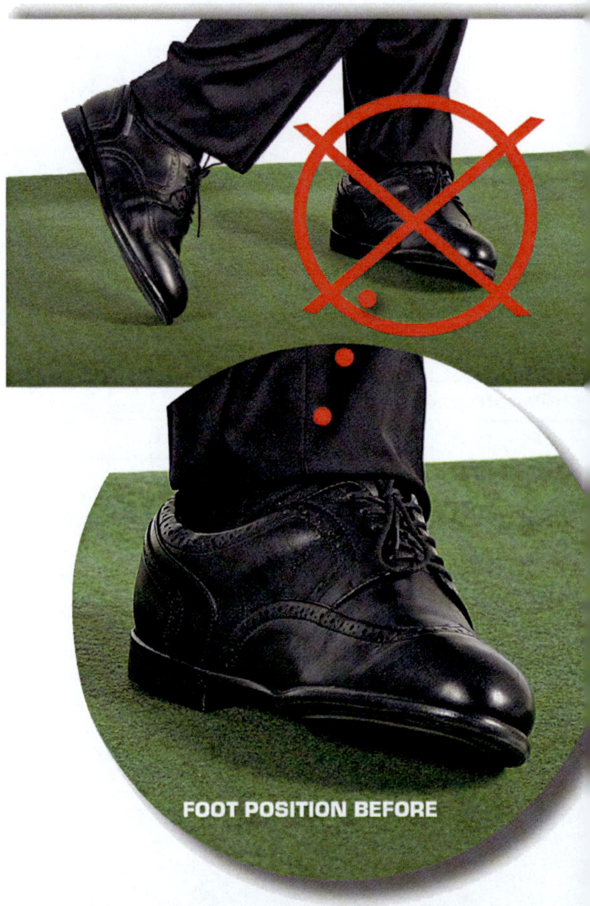

The Turning Shoe does not have any influence on performance because it only releases after ball impact.

(See below)

The Turning Shoe is suitable for any swing method.

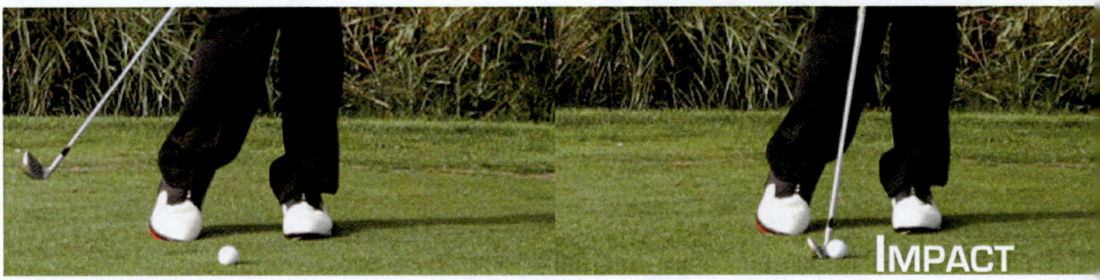

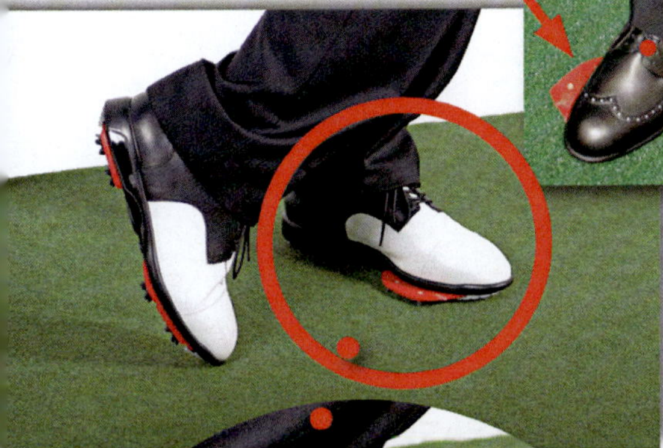

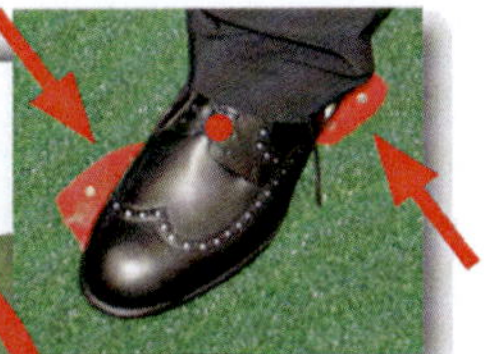

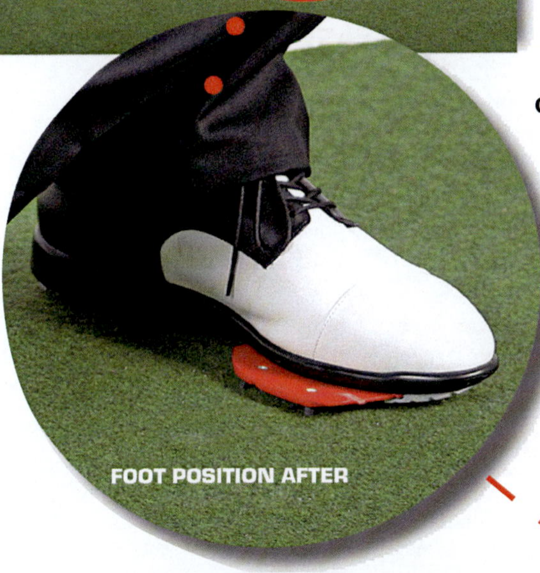

The Turning Shoe Health Promoter is the only golf shoe sole system which may be allowed for the Olympics and all tournaments according to the Rules of Golf, IOC Medical Code and the WORLD ANTI-DOPING AGENCY (WADA) CHARTER. It is the only system which promotes the golfer´s health during every single swing and reduces the risk of injury by a factor of 15. The Turning Shoe releases after ball impact and thus has no influence on the ball flight.

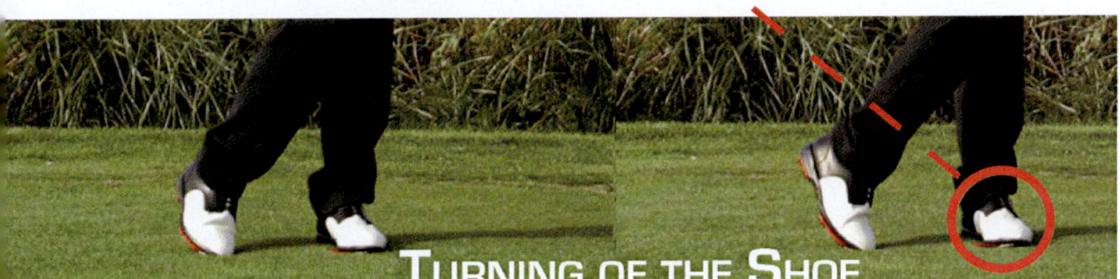

2.1. Health-Management with the Turning Shoe

Minimizing risk of injury from torsion

Twisting forces in the spine:	-99%
Twisting forces in the hip:	-89%
Twisting forces in the knee:	-99%
Twisting forces in the ankle:	-98%

These scientific results have been documented in a comprehensive investigative report with the accompanying derivations.

Reduction of pressure in Newton Meters (Nm) with and without the FREE-RELEASE® Golf Shoe.

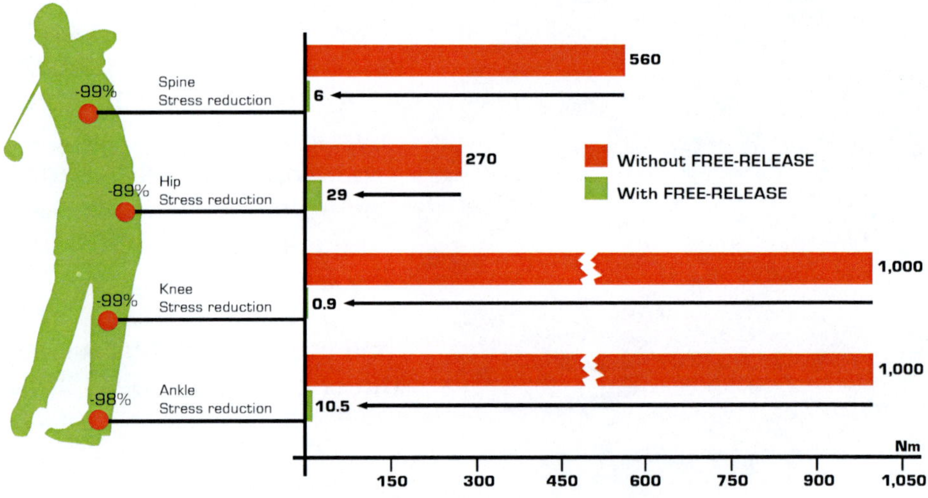

PGA Pro body weight 73 kg

“It is the
responsibility of

- Associations
- Golf instructors
- Functionaries
- Industry

to reduce the risk of
injury among all golfers
by a factor of

15! “

Frank Drollinger

3. Success with personal training

3.1. The "GOLF-PERSONAL-TRAINER" according to the Golf-Active-Method FREE-RELEASE®

Friends and acquaintances repeatedly tell me that they would like to start playing golf when they retire from working life. I cannot fully understand such statements, because golf is a fascinating sport for both young and old.

It is only important that a person has the necessary physical fitness in order to be able to execute a golf swing correctly.

You can monitor and define your personal fitness with lactate tests and performance diagnostics.

Our partner for this is Dr. Winfried Harer from the Herzklinik Ulm (Ulm Cardiology Clinic) in Germany.

However, based on my experience I know that general fitness training which is not aligned to the specific physical requirements

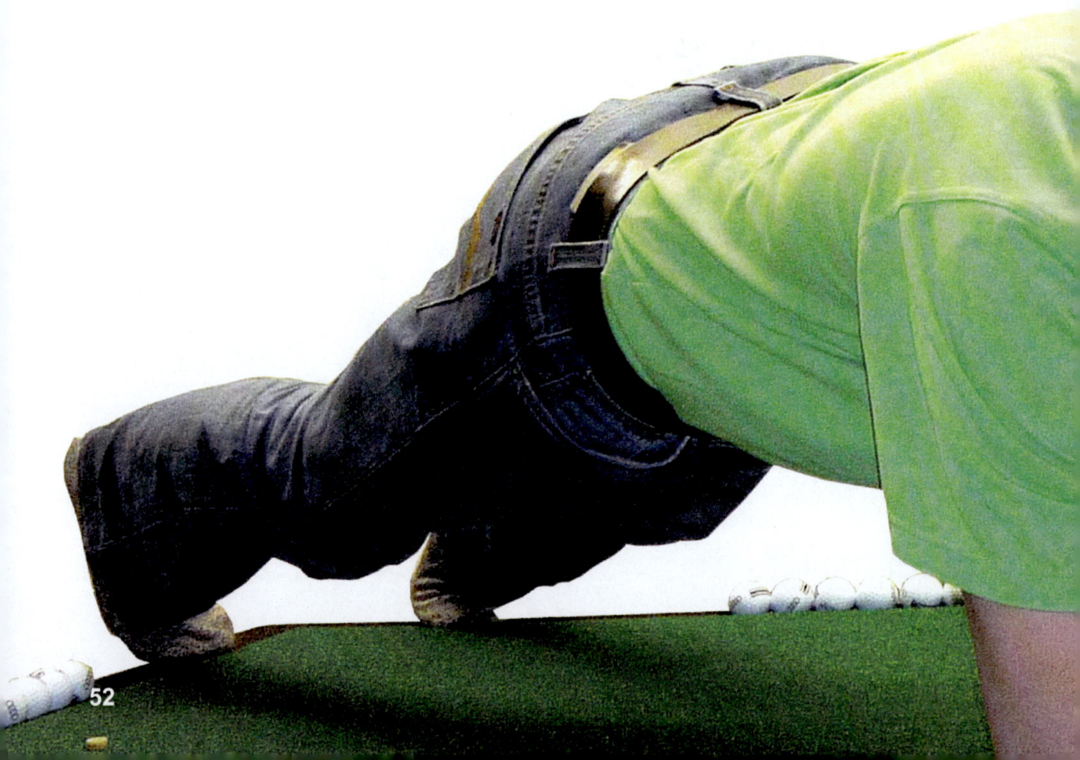

and problems of golf will bring you less benefit and success for your game.

That is why I have created a special training and fitness concept for golfers together with an appropriate educational program for fitness trainers known as

“GOLF-PERSONAL-TRAINER“.

With this specific fitness program the basic fitness will be strengthened, the flexibility and above all the particular motion will be practiced and combined with balance training in order to develop active legwork from passive legwork.

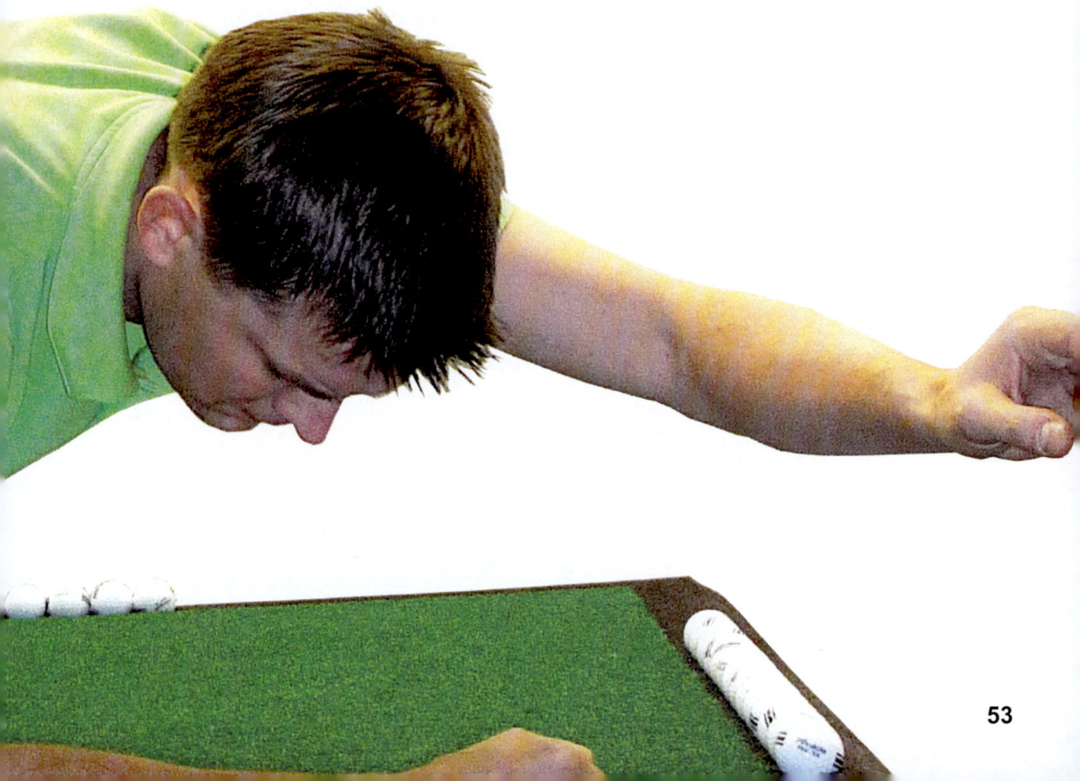

3.2. European Tour player Florian Fritsch

It was in January 2010 when I saw Florian for the first time in the lobby of Golf Club St. Leon-Rot. A few weeks later, in early March 2010, I learned from the media that Florian had announced his retirement from professional and competitive golf.

Even then it was clear that the performance pressure exerted on him by individuals in his athletic environment had been so great that he experienced enormous mental difficulties.

He told me that he had been removed from the developmental squad because he did not render the performance required to obtain a European Tour card. After that, he himself announced his retirement and indicated in numerous press interviews that he suffered from fear of flying.

Without further ado I called Florian and told him that I had analyzed video sequences of his swing beforehand and while doing so had detected that his swing at that time was perhaps good enough for first-class amateur golf, but by far not sufficient for a successful Tour career.

I explained to Florian that he was not to blame for his inadequate results for the Tour card, but he could not manage with the "outdated" swing motion. Florian has an extremely pronounced emotional intelligence and knows that he requires balance and active legwork in order to render sustainable performance and be able to hold his own on the Tour. The passive portions of his swing, i.e. energy transfer from the legs and hip/shoulder angle (X-factor 2) at the moment of impact were unsatisfactory for his possibilities.

Subsequent high-speed images proved it: Florian's legwork started only approx. 0.4 seconds after ball impact.

But Florian had problems with his hip due to torn diagonal abdominal muscles. The consequence of this passive legwork: the arms rolled over. The consequence of over-winding forearms is **no** repeatability of target precision.

I then explained to Florian that my team and me are always looking for talented competitive golfers.

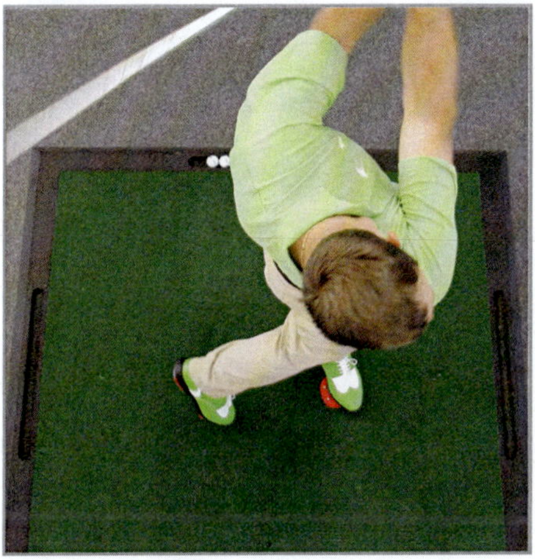

Shortly after the start of the FREE-RELEASE® training program we had already achieved such great motional advances in June 2010 that I decided to appoint Florian Fritsch as head of the GAM FREE-RELEASE® demo team.

Florian perceived this appointment as a great honor and assumed the managerial function in the demo team with considerable dedication and great enthusiasm.

Then Florian managed the great achievement in December. During his participation in the Q-School he prevailed against approx. 3,000 competitors and ultimately garnered a sixth place – and thereby a Tour card for 2011! From now on Florian will play alongside such prominent Tour pros as Martin Kaymer and Lee Westwood on the European Tour for the Race to Dubai.

Now I look forward to witnessing which path Florian's athletic career will take.

Unlike many other players, Florian does not require an extensive training workload. But he does need the right environment and natural kinematics. However, at the moment I am not so optimistic. Florian is already repeating the mistakes he once made.

Regular reference evaluations of the swing through myself and a member of our performance team at least twice a week are indispensable in order to provide Florian with feedback for possibly necessary fine corrections of his swing. Without consistent adherence to such a biomechanical and sports medicine training plan it may be difficult for Florian as well as any other Tour newcomer to sustainably assert themselves on the Tour.

In my professional assessment and in view of the by no means optimal swing quality of the Top 20 players on the US PGA Tour, Florian would have had the very best prospects of permanently establishing himself on the Tour.

The greatest danger of all for Tour players like Florian lies in their personal and business environment. If a player surrounds himself with dubious management or otherwise becomes dependent on people who only pursue their own interests, negative personal or business influences can very quickly lead to an athletic crash.

The swing training with Florian Fritsch makes one thing clear:

The Golf-Active-Method FREE-RELEASE® gets even "rejected" talents into gear.

We can significantly improve the performance of any golfer – amateurs as well as pros – with this method!

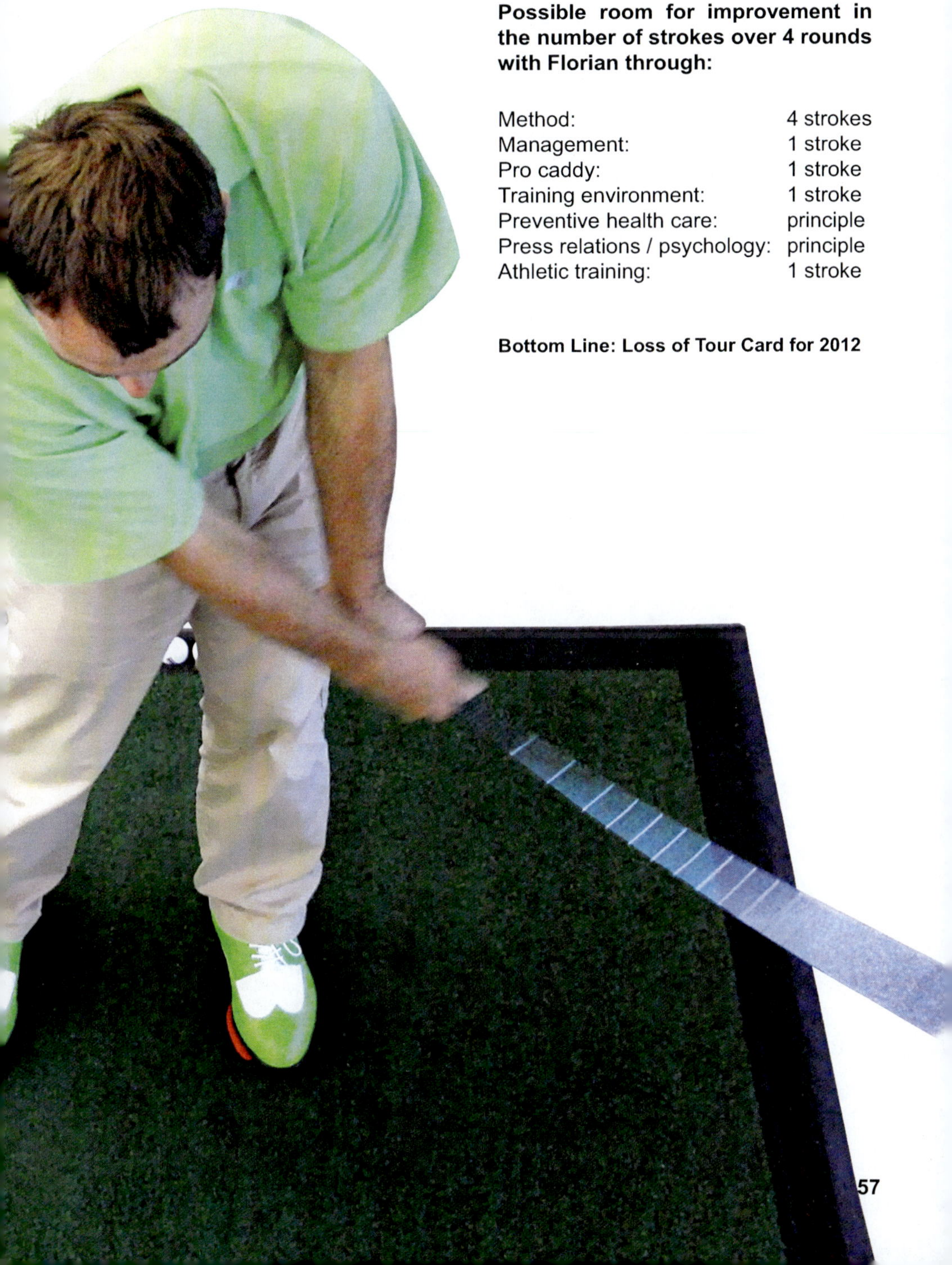

Possible room for improvement in the number of strokes over 4 rounds with Florian through:

Method:	4 strokes
Management:	1 stroke
Pro caddy:	1 stroke
Training environment:	1 stroke
Preventive health care:	principle
Press relations / psychology:	principle
Athletic training:	1 stroke

Bottom Line: Loss of Tour Card for 2012

3.2.a. Competitive ability of Tour players

The old golf swing method has reached its limits. Those who win are not the best golfers, but those who bear the highest risks of injury. This strategy is associated with a high risk. Today the modern Tour player must remember that short-term success and high health risk can also mean a short career.

The era of "circus horses" – i.e. Tour players who want to outwit the laws of anatomy, biomechanics and sports medicine – is coming to an end. Only those athletes who exclude all risks which can minimize their performance capability, who have a sustainable health management system at their disposal and apply repeatable biomechanics will achieve the successes necessary to obtain

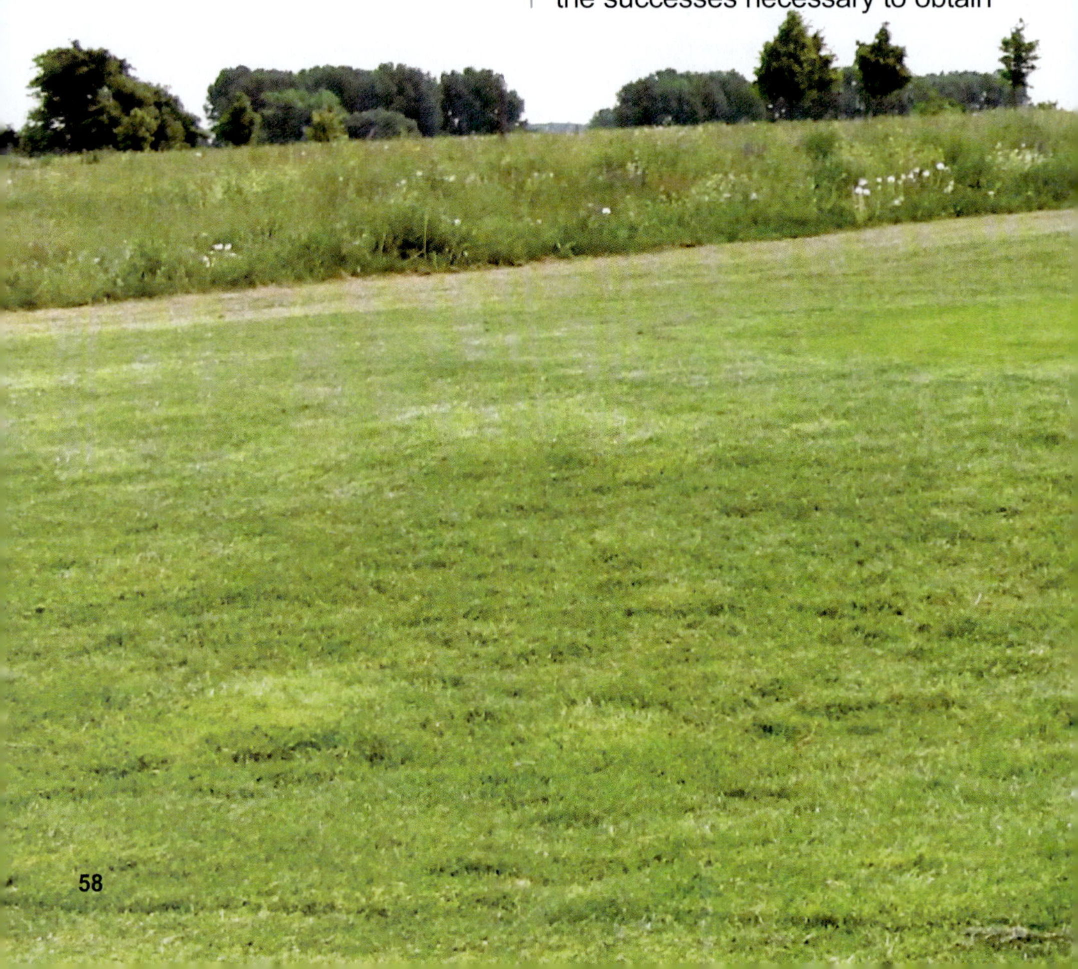

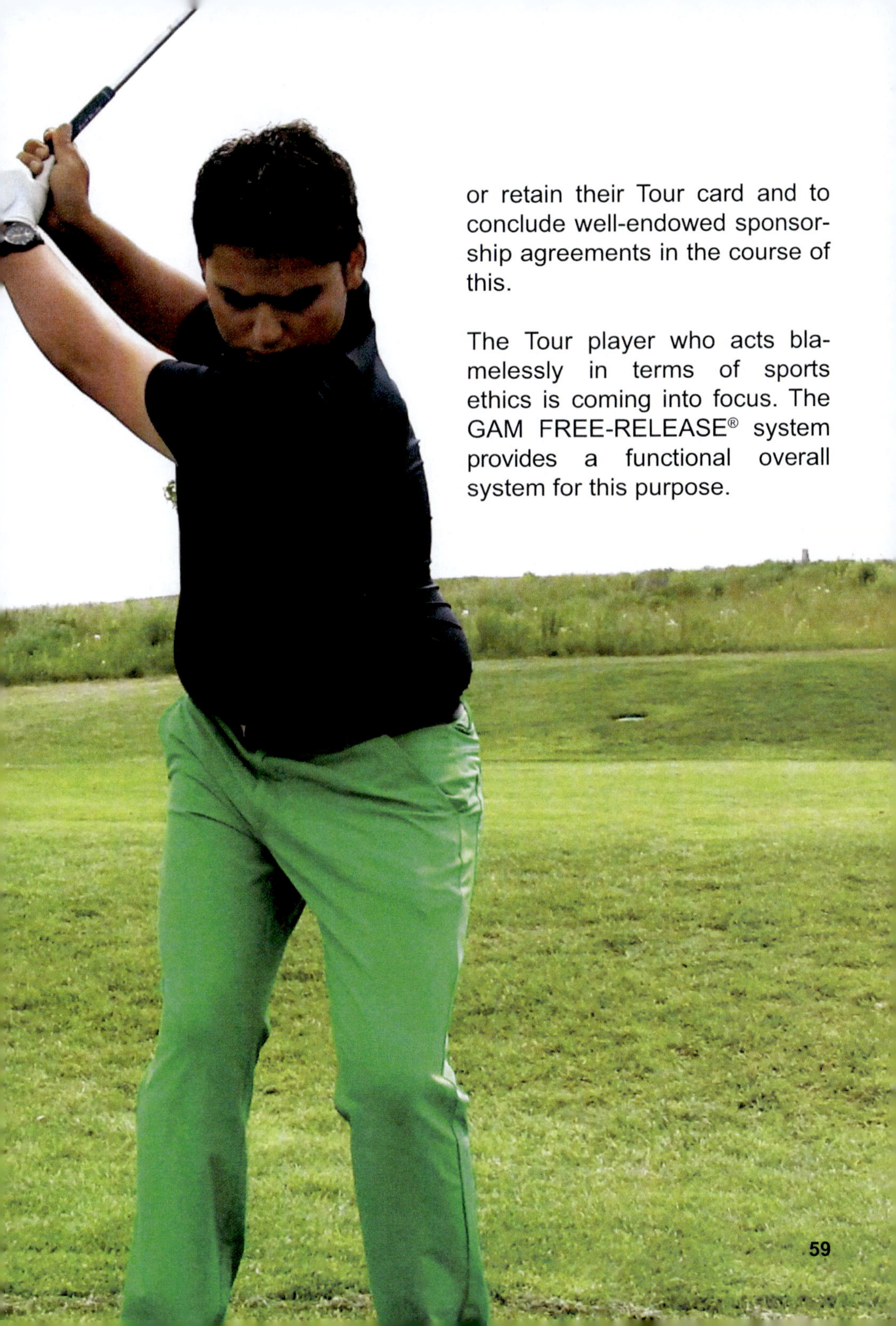

or retain their Tour card and to conclude well-endowed sponsorship agreements in the course of this.

The Tour player who acts blamelessly in terms of sports ethics is coming into focus. The GAM FREE-RELEASE® system provides a functional overall system for this purpose.

4. Golf swing methods

4.1. Method definition

The definition of a method in kinematics is in principle quite simple.

In golf the swing is divided into so-called "main swing sequences". The structure is comparable with a pie.

The individual slices of the pie can be described with the individual main functional phases of the swing. A main functional phase differs from a swing variation in that the athlete cannot do without this part of the overall motion in order to execute an entire swing.

If it is possible to replace a main function with another main function, it is said that a new swing method is created.

Ben Hogan, whom I highly regard, broke down the golf swing into so-called "main functional phases" in approx. 1950.

The swing descriptions of the well-known golf and teaching association books all paraphrase the same main functional phases.

After 60+ years I have managed to modify, replace or improve some of Ben Hogan's main functional phases. My method is called "Golf-Active-Method FREE- RELEASE®", or simply "FREE-RELEASE®".

The advantages of my FREE-RELEASE-Method® lie in the following areas:

- Health, i.e. minimization of the risk of injury by a factor of 15
- Improvement of the transfer of energy to the ball
- Acceleration of learning progress by a factor of 4
- Improvement of ball impact
- Improved repeatability of good strokes

Examples for the replacement of individual main functional phases:

1. **Setup balance *instead of*** setup position in imbalance and without axis parallelism.

2. **Backswing balance *instead of*** transition with shifting of weight to the backswing foot.

3. **Active legwork,** i.e. big toe joint deliberately initiates the downswing in a rotational push in order to utilize muscle power to accelerate the hip by approx. 67 degrees towards the ball impact and then towards the target – ***instead of*** a blockade of the right leg muscles, i.e. the arms initiate the downswing; the legwork follows suit and does not have any energetic influence on the ball impact.

4.2. Difference between a method and the variation of a method

What is the difference between a method and a mere variation in the sphere of kinematics?

This question is only seemingly insignificant. It is actually symptomatic of one of the main problems in golf:

The technically and scientifically insufficient qualification of participants in teaching activities, starting with golf instructors in the local golf club and including the universally well-known and highly revered 'trainer gurus'.

The golf instructor is more victim than "culprit" in this context.

In a conversation with one of these 'great trainers' he was of the opinion that he did not even teach the Ben Hogan method at all.

When asked afterwards about which method he did teach, he answered that he instructed according to the PGA model. This aroused my interest and I asked my conversation partner to explain which main functions of the PGA model differ from the Ben Hogan method.

The trainer explained that he knew nothing about it, and that he had no idea of how a method can be defined.

A bit later he added that he feels uneasy in such technical discussions because he would usually made a poor impression in this connection.

But this is not about who looks better or worse in technical discussions. This is about facts, facts which lead to improvements.

I actually believe that the technical exchange – just like research and development – should solely have the purpose of increasing knowledge and promoting progressive solutions.

A method consists of indispensable main motion functions

Ben Hogan Method

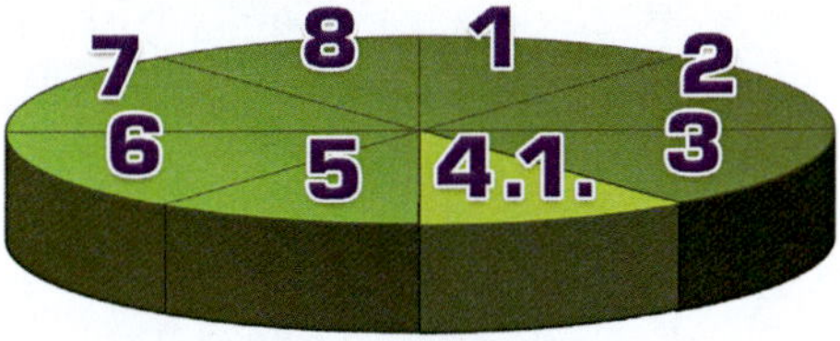

Frank Drollinger Method

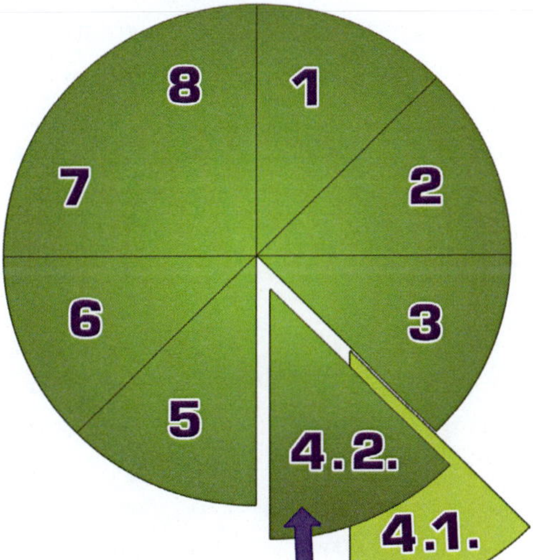

I replaced seven main functions with functions that are appreciably improved in terms of energy and sports medicine. This is the sports science justification that I have managed to create a new method.

In practically all areas of everyday life – including sports – we have witnessed rapid technical development: what started in the realm of telecommunications with smoke signals, progressed into telegraphs and the first telephone continues in the presentday smartphone.

There is no sensible reason why technical development should not take place in golf. But instead, traditional technique – in the form of the swing method developed by Ben Hogan, which gathered dust for over 60 years – is retained.

In particular, it is also regarded as proven fact that the method of Ben Hogan generates untenable torsional loads.

Golf is a sport in which traditions are maintained. But the awareness of tradition and progressiveness are not mutually exclusive. Quite the contrary! Like other sports, golf is also dependent on new technical and methodical impulses in order to win future generations for this traditional sport. My sports science expertise in the field of methodology is based on the models from Prof. Dr. Ulrich Göhner, University of Tübingen. Like no other researcher, Göhner broke down and analyzed the motion sequences of various sports disciplines into their individual motional components.

I became sensitized to this model during my 20+ year career. Added to this is the fact that based on my many years of experience in sport supervision I developed a special talent for motion sequences and seeing mistakes. Acquiring knowledge of classic mechanics also helped me to gain a profound understanding of the overall system of golf biomechanics.

Back to the methodologies of Prof. Dr. Göhner: the totality of the motion sequence is to be initially considered for evaluation of the methodical autonomy of a motion technique.

In the next step, the motion sequence is separated into segments, so-called “main functional phases”. According to Göhner, this merely involves a variation if optical motional modifications are made in the framed segments of the motion sequence which do not pertain to the main functions and consequently do not bring about any fundamental change of the overall motion sequence.

In contrast, according to the system from Göhner, a method is to be referred to as new and autonomous if main functions of a motion sequence are replaced or removed.

I have made precisely such modifications during the further development of the Ben Hogan method into the Golf-Active-Method FREE-RELEASE®. In particular, the following differences ensue between the GAM FREE-RELEASE® and the conventional swing according to Ben Hogan:

- **Measurable balance in the setup position**
- **Shifting of weight in the backswing is omitted**
- **Active, controlled shoulder rotation in the backswing**
- **The body's center of gravity is almost fixed during the swing phase B1**
- **The rotational axis is nearly fixed during the swing-phase B1**
- **Active instead of passive leg and hip work**
- **Active, controlled rotational impulse in the downswing, released by means of the right big toe joint**
- **The active rotational impulse accelerates actively the hip from the starting point X-factor 1 to 2 by approx. 67.5 degrees**
- **No composite motion from lateral hip thrust and body rotation, but stable rotation around a nearly fixed base axis**
- **Actively controlled hip rotation, physiologically implemented, i.e. without torsional load in the lumbar spine**
- **In the follow-through and finish there is no rotation over the hip, knee & ankle joint of the target leg, and no supination and no influence of force on the ankle joint**

- **Healthy overall motion pattern; previously common influences of force in the form of shearing forces, friction, torsion, pressure on the intervertebral discs and vibration are reduced by up to 99%**

The overall motion pattern of the Ben Hogan method can be described as the "Double Pendulum Thrust Passive Rotation Method".

I describe the **Ben Hogan method briefly** as the **"Passive Method"**, whereas in contrast to this I describe the Golf-Active-Method FREE-RELEASE® as the **"Single Pendulum Active Rotation Method"** and consequently as the **"Active Method"**.

According to sports science and sports medicine standards, GAM FREE-RELEASE® is the first new swing method since Ben Hogan described his method of golf swing.

As a result, GAM FREE-RELEASE® assumes the function of the new control technique in the realm of golf.

Every physics student learns in their first semester that a thrust-rotational motion can never be as efficient as a fixed rotational motion.

These physiologically and energetically optimal values cannot be achieved with any other method than GAM FREE-RELEASE®.

stress-free finish position for the spine

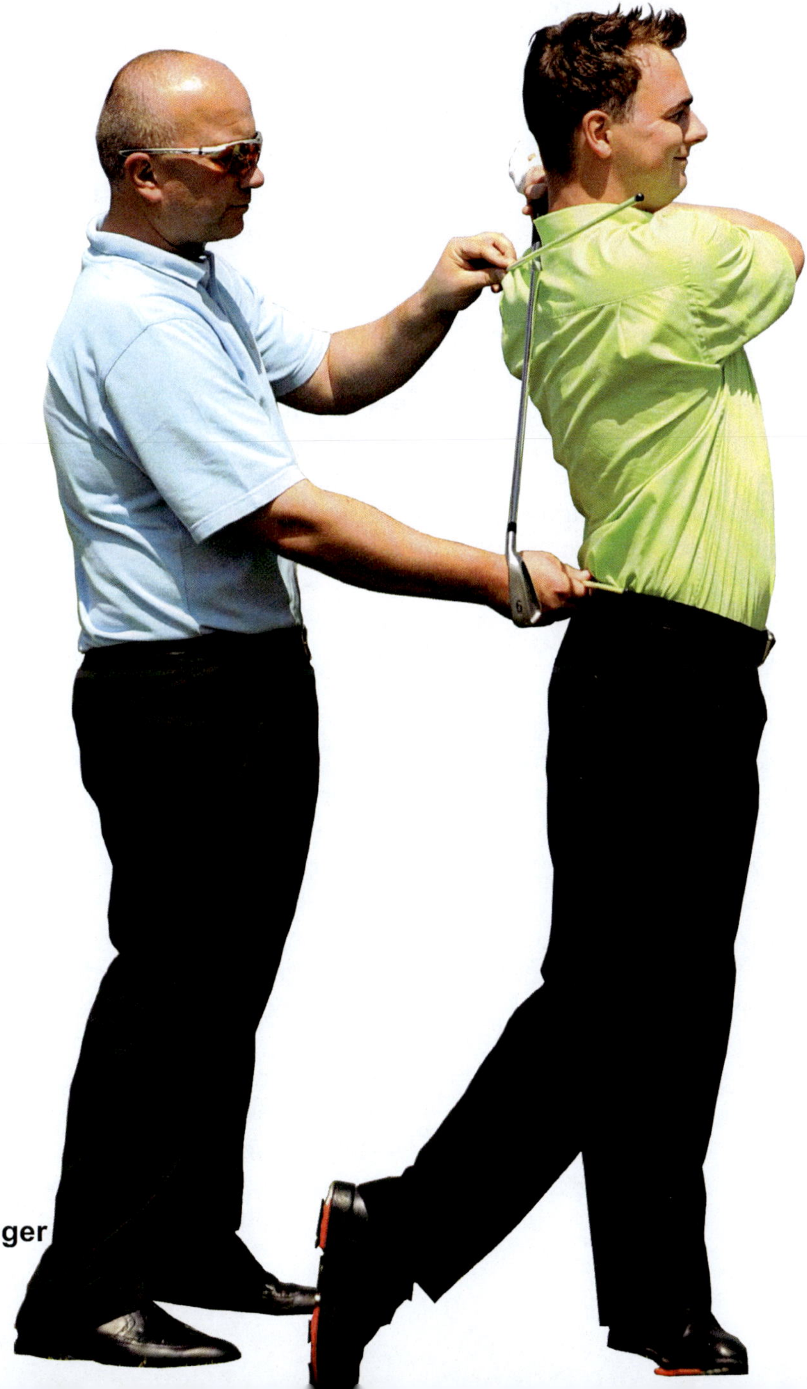

Frank Drollinger

4.3. Method comparison: Ben Hogan & Golf-Active-Method FREE-RELEASE®

According to the method definition, there are actually only two golf swing methods:

Ben Hogan approx. 1950
Frank Drollinger 2010

We also found another 'half-method' called "Stack & Tilt", but this will not be elaborated on for reasons of clarity.

The method I have developed makes unnatural motions natural. Up until now, we had to take a wide stance with the method according to Ben Hogan.

A disadvantageous consequence of this wide stance was that the hip rotation in the

X-factor 1-2-3

I defined myself was reduced to a harmful +45 degrees instead of the biomechanically ideal +90 degrees. The pelvis was torn towards the target via the diagonal abdominal muscles.

In contrast, GAM FREE-RELEASE® makes hip rotation easier due to a narrower stance, whereby it is much easier for the golfer to implement a biomechanically optimal motion.

Whereas the muscles of the backswing leg are blocked in their activity due to the weight shift and the body falls into a state of imbalance during the golf swing according to the Ben Hogan model, with GAM FREE-RELEASE® the golfer is in a state of measurable balance during the swing phase from backswing until the ball impact.

Only in such a state of body balance is it even possible to employ the large muscle groups of the backswing leg actively and rationally so that the energy from a hip acceleration path of approx. 67.5 degrees can be additionally transferred to the golf ball.

It is also important that the target precision is substantially increased through an active hip acceleration. Whereas the body's center of gravity (COG) during a golf swing according to the Ben Hogan method is so-called "hypermobile" (approx. 14 cm) until the moment of impact, the GAM FREE-RELEASE® measurements in the swing phase until ball impact show an almost completely fixed COG of approx. 3 cm.

The fixation of COG – i.e. the prevention of weight shifts in the backswing until ball impact – is an indispensable prerequisite for being able to implement a reproducible ball-club head impact angle under 2.5 degrees.

Another methodical improvement is that the numerous passive – i.e. not consciously rational – motion elements of the swing according to Ben Hogan will be transformed into active, i.e. deliberately induced, swing elements during the GAM FREE-RELEASE®.

Compensatory motions – which are to be classified as unavoidable, but nevertheless as motion errors because of the inco sistent biomechanics of the swing according to Ben Hogan – will also become superfluous with the overall biomechanical functionality of motion sequences during the swing according to GAM FREE-RELEASE®.

The motion enables an improved transfer of energy to the golf ball, greater target precision and significantly increases the repeatability of this enhanced ball impact quality.

GAM FREE-RELEASE® can be divided into two blocks:

Block 1: Health protection, prophylaxis and therapy with hardware and software.

Block 2: Performance improvement in the sphere of energy transfer and precision through biomechanical optimization of motion sequences.

In summary, the differences in the

individual swing phases between the Ben Hogan method and the FREE-RELEASE-Method® can be depicted as follows:

Setup:

An imbalance prevails with the Ben Hogan method; the right foot is burdened; an imbalance in the setup position complicates the flow of motion; the result is a lateral pelvic motion and a hypermobile COG.

That is why we speak about a “double pendulum thrust-thrust rotation swing” (body and arms “swing back and forth”). FREE-RELEASE® is a “single pendulum rotary swing”.

With the Ben Hogan method there is no parallel standing position of feet, knees and hip. As a result, compromises in the alignment will be made, i.e. the target precision suffers and will be particularly difficult to implement.

Backswing:

The backswing with the Ben Hogan method starts in the left shoulder.

In contrast, the backswing of the Frank Drollinger FREE-RELEASE-Method® starts at three points: back of the left hand, right hip and right shoulder.

In the Ben Hogan method we find a lateral hip thrust with a clear weight shift to the backswing foot.

The right leg muscles will be “sandwiched” and “blocked” because of this.

FREE-RELEASE® turns on its own body axis in measureable balance. As a result, the large right leg muscles are “able to work”.

FREE-RELEASE®: the left upper arm is pressed against the chest and serves as a “guide”; the backswing path occurs in sync with the hip rotation up to 45 degrees.

The club shaft intersects the right shoulder axis. Foregoing the lateral “planing away” across the right hip joint enables significant protection of the articular cartilage there. The right outer (lateral) meniscus is also spared.

Downswing:
The downswing in the Ben Hogan method is initiated through a shoulder/arm rotation and indentation of the inner edge of the right foot.

The diagonal abdominal muscles turn the pelvis towards the target. This muscle group enables approx. 50 watts at peak. Active legwork enables approx. 1,000 watts.

With the Ben Hogan method this leads to a further lateral thrust (planing away of the left hip joint cartilage and knee joint cartilage). The arms swing faster than the legwork; at the time of impact it is impossible that energy is transferred from the leg muscles to the ball.

With FREE-RELEASE® the downswing is initiated via the big toe joint. The leg muscles are slower than the arms. The path of the shoulder is longer than that of the hip. Ideally, the pelvis is accelerated through the large leg muscles from the finish position until ball impact by approx. 67.5 degrees.

(all descriptions refer to a right hander)

4.3.a. Comparison of Method Concept

Principle of the body's center of gravity during the set-up, backswing phases up to ball impact

BEN HOGAN METHOD

METHOD CONCEPT:
BODY'S CENTER OF GRAVITY TRACES DIAGONAL „8"

(Shift in body's center of gravity would not be intended by target athletes, e.g. sports marksmen, who emphasize target precision and hit rate.)

Hypermobile center of gravity

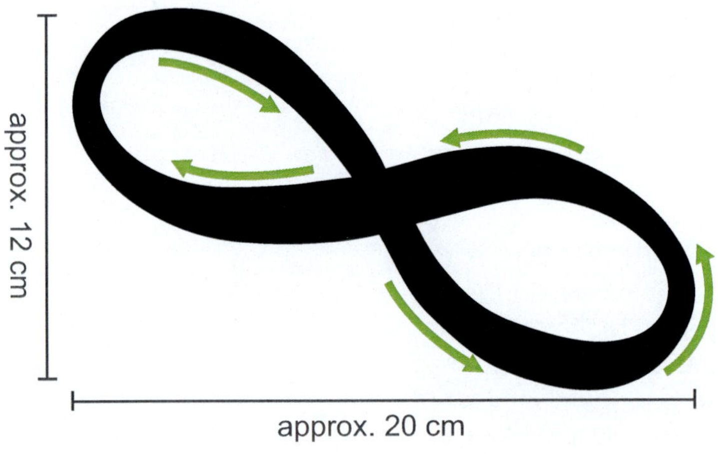

Scale: 1:2,5

FRANK DROLLINGER FREE-RELEASE-METHOD®

METHOD CONCEPT:
FIXATION OF BODY'S CENTER OF GRAVITY INSOFAR AS POSSIBLE DURING THE SET-UP AND BACKSWING PHASES UP TO BALL IMPACT

"Target-Sport-Quality"

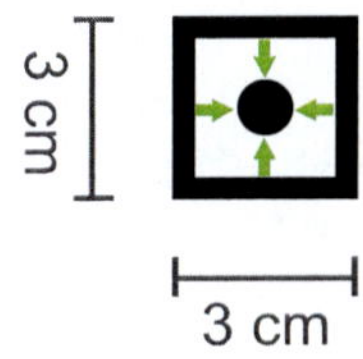

Scale: 1:2,5

4.4. Olympic requirement for a healthy method

The members of the Olympic Movement guarantee that the safety conditions and medical care will benefit the physical and mental health of athletes.

The members of the Olympic Movement must take all necessary measures to achieve this goal and to minimize the athlete's risks of injury and illness.

Golf loses its meaning and its attraction without respect for rules.

The winner at present is not the best athlete, but the participant who is willing to take the greatest health risks in order to win.

Whoever accepts the greatest health risks in order to win – and an already injured golfer acts exactly in this manner – violates the fundamental principles of the spirit of the game as well as the IOC Charter.

According to the Rules of Golf, an injured player may not participate in a tournament and must even discontinue his or her training.

The IOC communicates with the respective umbrella organizations. In golf this is the International Golf Federation (IGF). Since 2011 the IGF has maintained an office at the IOC's headquarters in Lausanne, Switzerland. The associations are sensitized to the topic "health protection of athletes" and nurtured with regard to compliance with regulations through the exchange and cooperation among the individual umbrella organizations. The IGF and its 143 national associations must make up ground for 50 years of lack of action. We have performed the majority of this work for the IGF. As an item of health protection equipment similar to the helmet in alpine skiing, the Turning Shoe Health Promoter merely has to provide this impetus. As a result, the sport of golf demonstrates that it is willing to comply with the statutory obligations of the Olympics, World Anti-Doping Agency (WADA) and the Rules of Golf.

The Golf-Active-Method FREE-RELEASE® system complies with the IGF, IOC and WADA requirements!

Extract from the Rules of Golf

- Rules of Golf are designed to care about the health of golfers respecting state-of-the-art findings in the field of sports medicine, focusing not only on the fact that players are not allowed to injure other players, but also the reverse conclusion is true that athletes should be allowed to do their utmost to reduce the risk of injuries while playing golf.

- IOC–Medical Code and Rule 7.1 of the IOC Charta:

"No practice constituting any form of physical injury or physiological harm to athletes is permissible."

- Purpose of the WADA to pursue health promotion including the reverse conclusion meaning that it is not only prohibited to use illegal drugs but also to allow athletes to do their utmost to protect their health which means for golfers to reduce stress, torsion, shearing force, friction, and pressure.

(Excerpt from IOC Medical Charta)

Chapter II: Protection and Promotion of the Athletes' Health during Training and Competition

7. General Principles

7.1. No practice constituting any form of physical injury or psychological harm to athletes should be acceptable.
Members of the Olympic Movement should ensure that the athletes' conditions of safety, well-being and medical care are favourable to their physical and mental equilibrium. They should adopt the necessary measures to achieve this end and to minimise the risk of injuries and illness. The participation of sports physicians is desirable in the drafting of such measures.

7.2. In each sports discipline, minimal safety requirements should be defined and applied with a view to protecting the health of the participants and the public during training and competition. Depending on the sport and the level of competition, specific rules should be adopted regarding sports venues, safe environmental conditions, sports equipment authorised or prohibited, and the training and competition programmes. The specific needs of each athlete category should be identified and respected.

7.3. For the benefit of all concerned, measures to safeguard the health of the athletes and to minimise the risks of physical injury and psychological harm should be publicised for the benefit all concerned.

7.4. Measures for the protection and the promotion of the athletes' health should be based on the latest recognised medical knowledge.

7.5. Research in sports medicine and sports sciences is encouraged and should be conducted in accordance with the recognised principles of research ethics, in particular the Declaration of Helsinki adopted by the World Medical Association (last revised in Seoul, 2008), and the applicable law. It must never be conducted in a manner which could harm an athlete's health or jeopardise his or her performance. The voluntary and informed consent of the athletes to participate in such research is essential.

5. Golf-Active-Method FREE-RELEASE®

5.1. Sequential description of golf swing motion

Swing sequence 1: Setup

1. 50/50 weight distribution on the left and right foot
2. Classic grip: the right thumb with the index finger placed in the middle of the grip forms a "V"; the grip is of great importance in the GAM!
3. Parallel foot position
4. Axis parallelism: foot, knee, hip and shoulder axis
5. Hand's width distance to the club grip
6. Attach great importance to the "alignment" (towards the target)

Sequential description

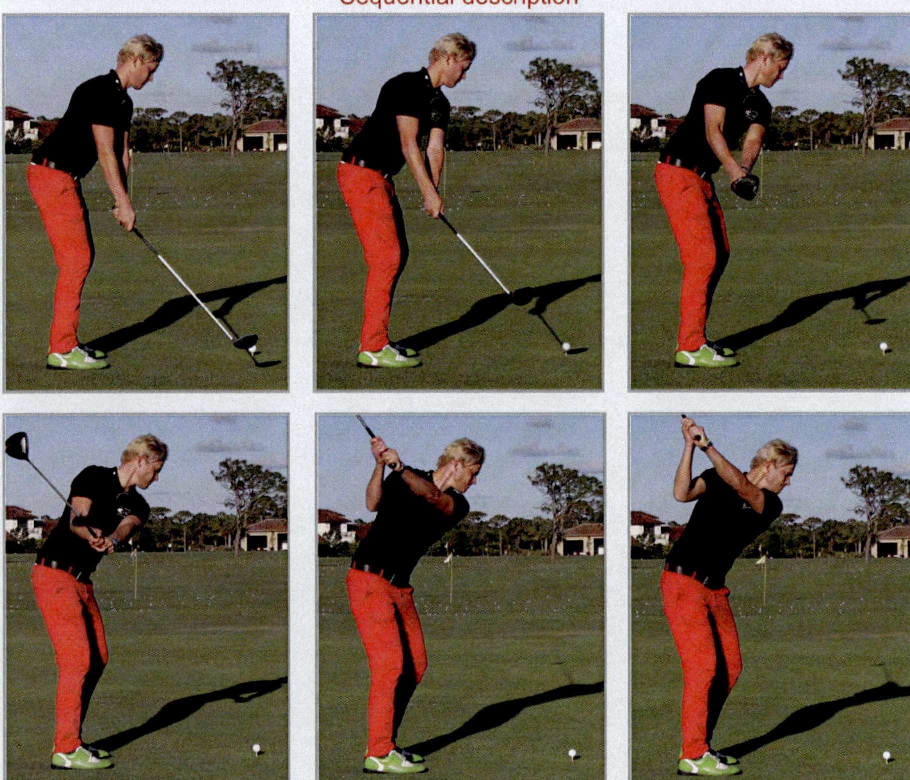

A student of Frank Drollinger: PGA PRO Eric Blomqvist, Sweden

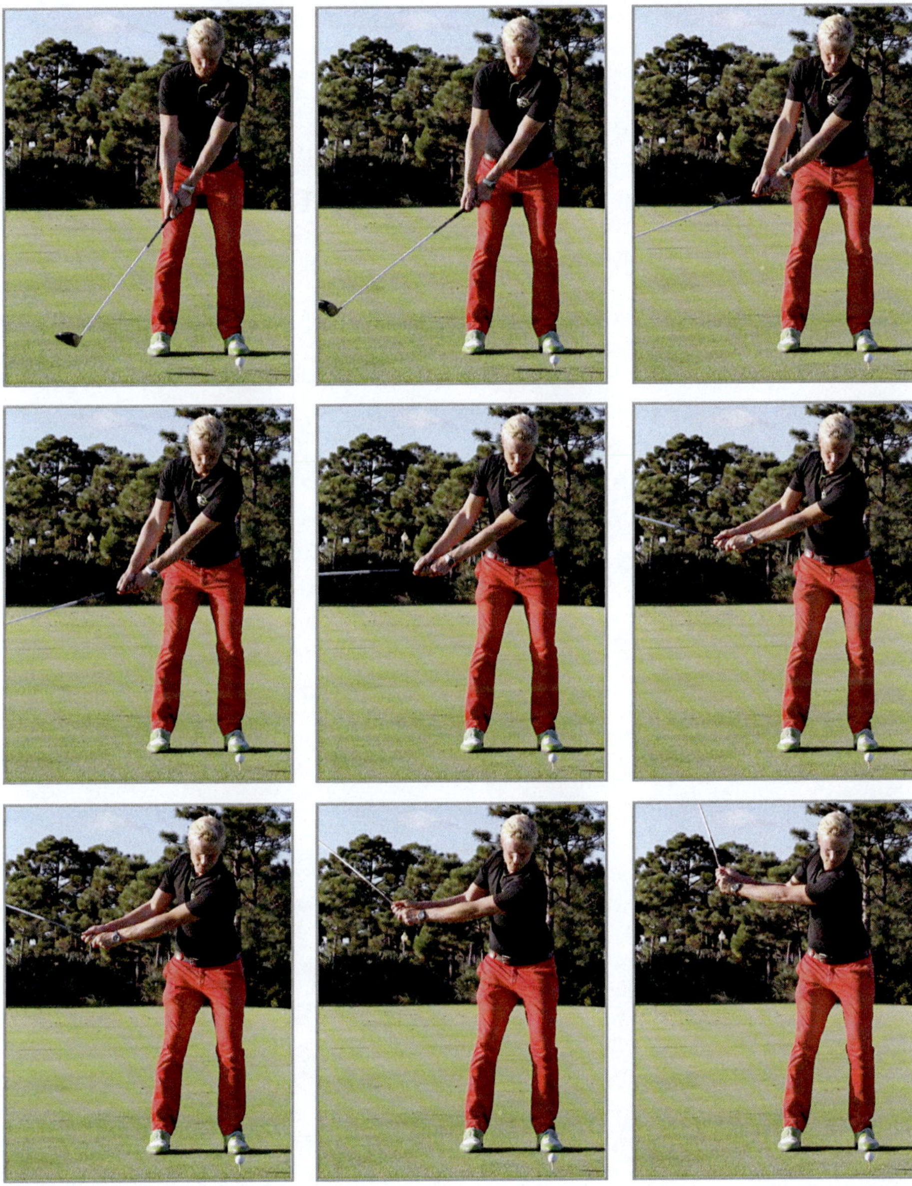

5.2. Golf-Active-Method FREE-RELEASE® fundamentals

What is balance, setup balance & backswing balance?

Setup balance

- Alignment towards the target (Fig. 1+5)
- Feet parallel (Fig. 2)
- Body weight 50:50 (Fig. 3)
- Shoes synchronous in length (Fig. 2)
- Knees parallel (Fig. 1+3)
- Hip parallel (Fig. 1+3)
- Shoulders parallel (Fig. 1+3)
- Chin as high as possible so that the shoulder has space and balance can be retained (Fig. 1)
- Knees bent in sync (Fig. 1)
- Upper body is bent between 35 and 40 degrees; can vary individually, i.e. depending on body stature (Fig. 1)
- Thigh bent at approx. 28 degrees (Fig.1)
- Pelvis backwards (Fig. 1)
- Back and head are one line (Fig.1)
- Distance to end of club is one hand's width (Fig. 1)
- Eyes parallel; head straight (Fig. 6)
- Grip: place the left hand slightly diagonal to the back of the hand; the right hand shows a "V" on the grip with "long" thumb and index finger (Fig. 4)
- Width of stance so that the right leg can actively move the right hip towards the target "horizon", i.e. left knee and right knee should be at a 90-degree angle in the finish (Fig. 6)
- Gluteal and thigh muscles are activated in this connection (Fig. 4)
- Centered club grip (Fig. 4)
- Centered ball position (Fig. 2) (Exception: ball is teed-up; driver, 3-wood (Fig. 3)).

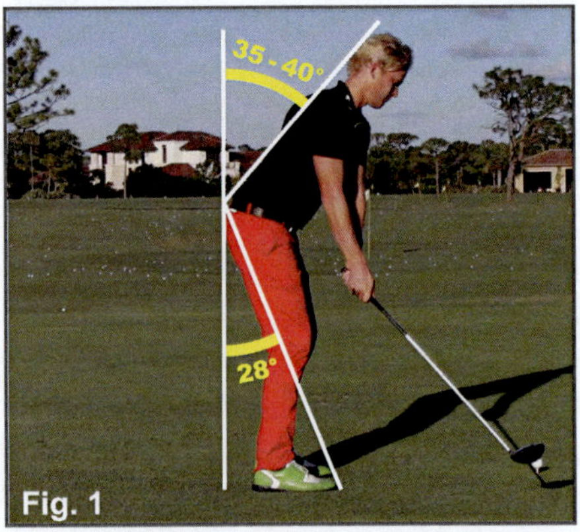

Fig. 1

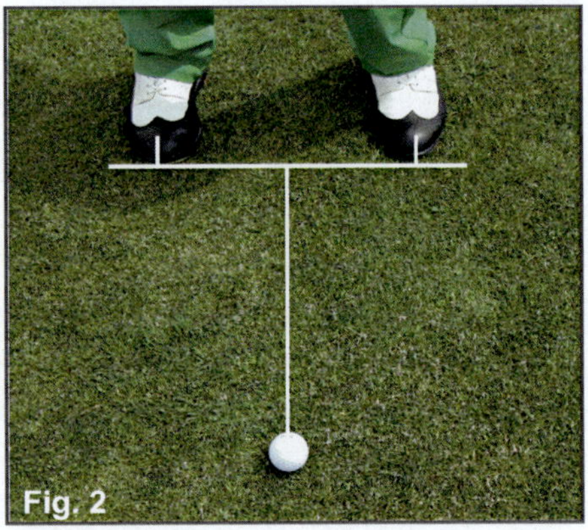
Fig. 2

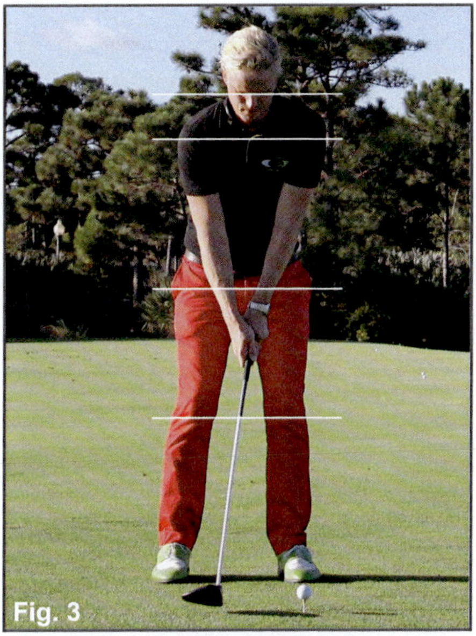

Fig. 3

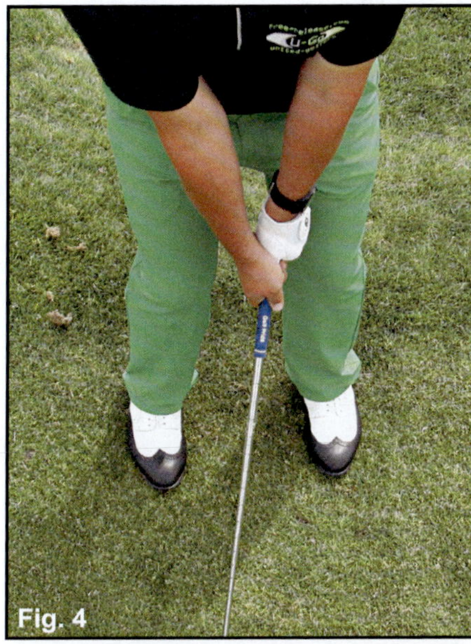

Fig. 4

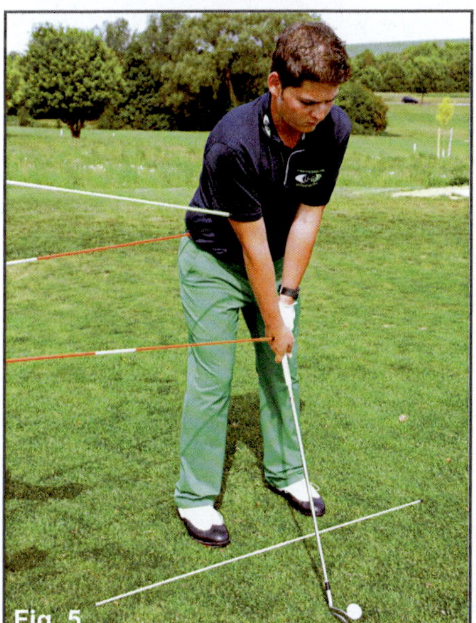

Fig. 5

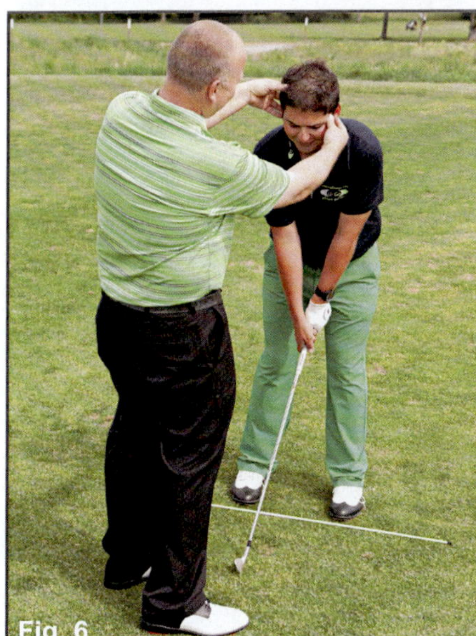

Fig. 6

Backswing balance

- The backswing is performed as a rotation around one's own central axis, "neutral axis" (Fig. 3)
- 3 points initiate the backswing synchronously and dynamically parallel to hip rotation: right hip, right shoulder, back of the left hand
- In this connection, the shoulder has the highest rotational speed and covers twice the path in relation to the hip; ideally 90 degrees (Fig. 1, see also Fig. 5+9)

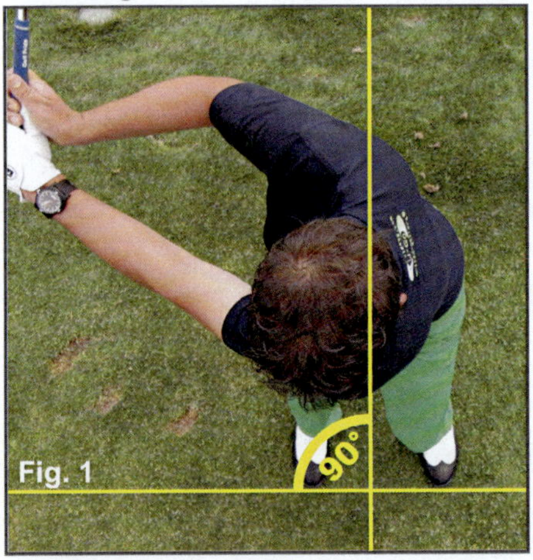

Fig. 1

- "Y" formed by arms and club; coordinated backswing speed (Fig. 13)
- The overall backswing tempo remains "steady", but deliberate; the goal in this connection is to keep the body's center of gravity and the balance "fixed" throughout the backswing (Fig. 2+3)
- Right knee remains absolutely bent! (Fig. 4)
- Left knee remains bent! (Fig. 4)
- Hip turns maximum 45 degrees (Fig. 5)
- Left foot remains stable on the ground (Fig. 2+3)
- Hip remains parallel to the ground throughout the backswing rotation (Fig. 3)
- Both arms together with the club form a "Y"; this "Y" is thrust in sync with the hip rotation so that the back of the left hand does not turn (Fig. 6)
- After this "Y" reaches the position of the outer right thigh, the left wrist is bent upward
- Left arm remains stretched (Fig. 4)
- Shaft intersects the right shoulder joint and in this connection has a parallel track in relation to the ball setup (Fig. 7)
- Standing weight remains 50:50, i.e. in measurable balance (Fig. 2+3)
- End of backswing: the club shaft is positioned maximally parallel to the ground (Fig. 2+3)

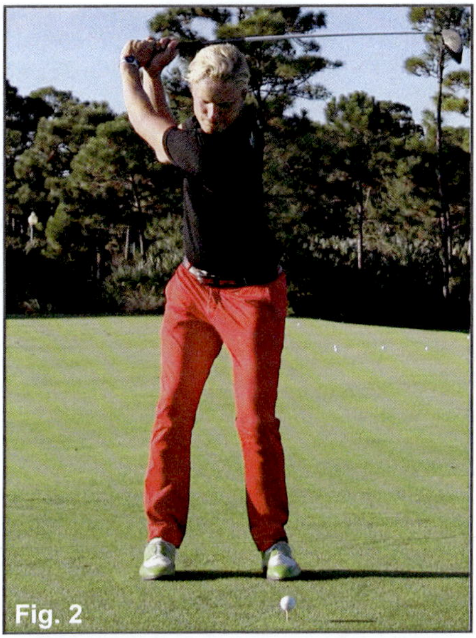
Fig. 2

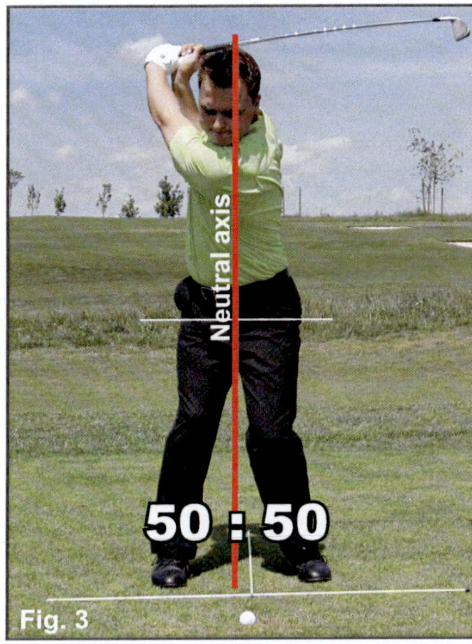

Fig. 3

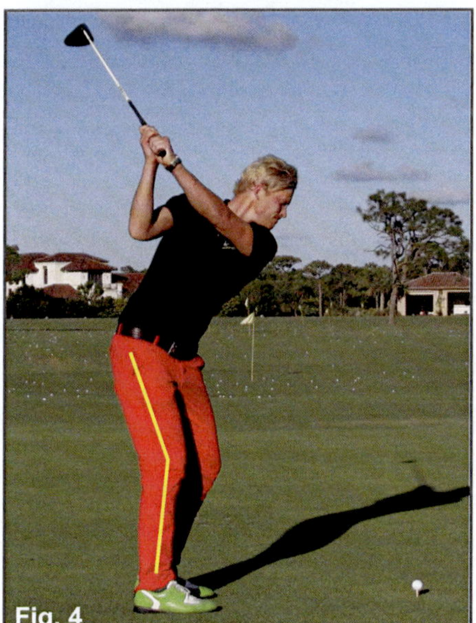
Fig. 4

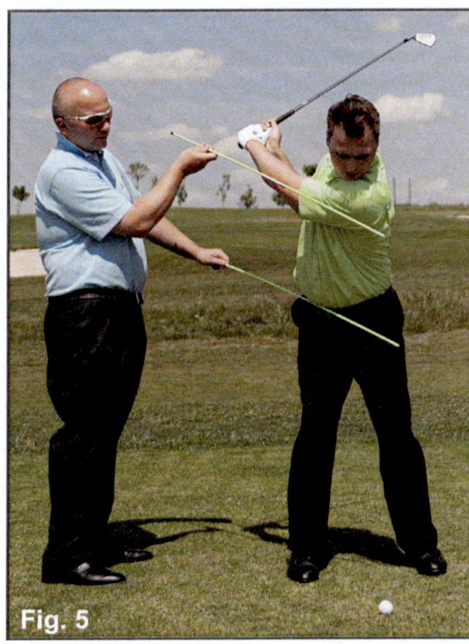
Fig. 5

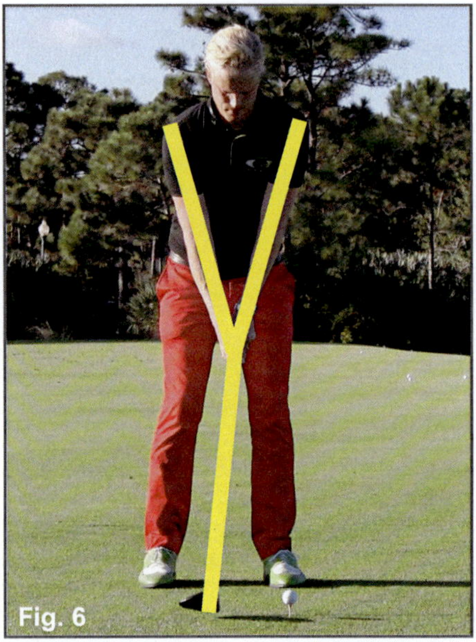

Fig. 6

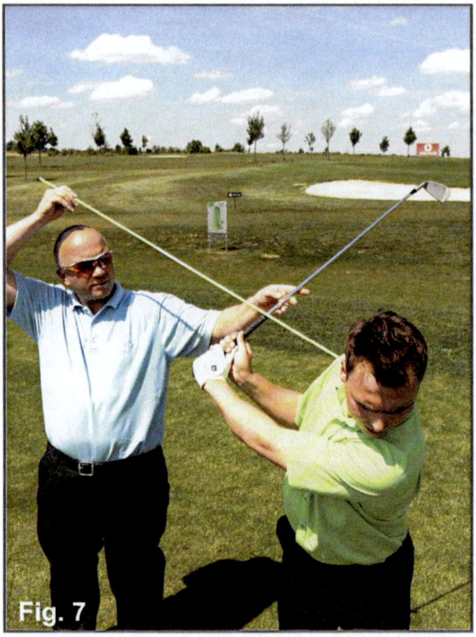

Fig. 7

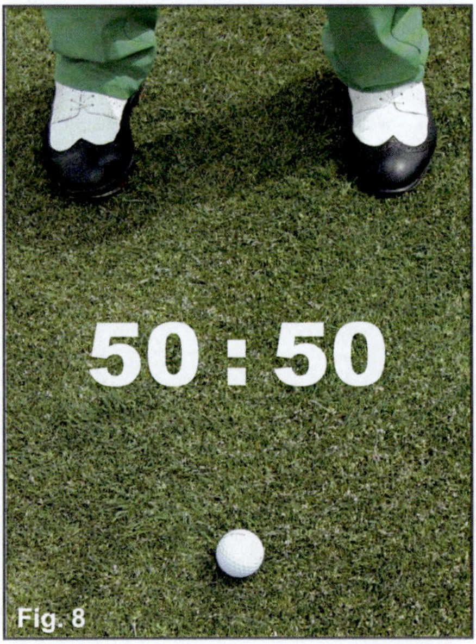

Fig. 8

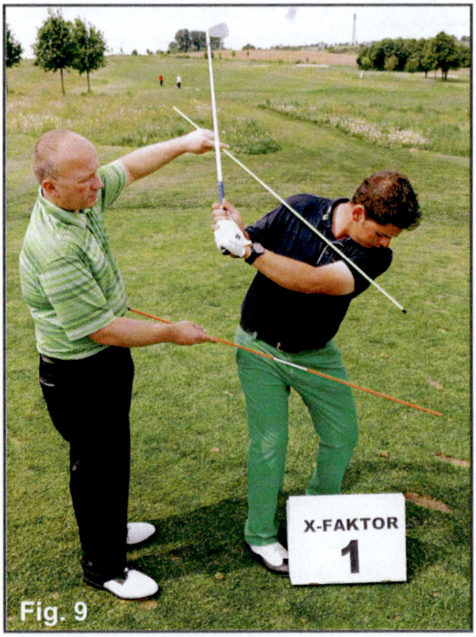

Fig. 9

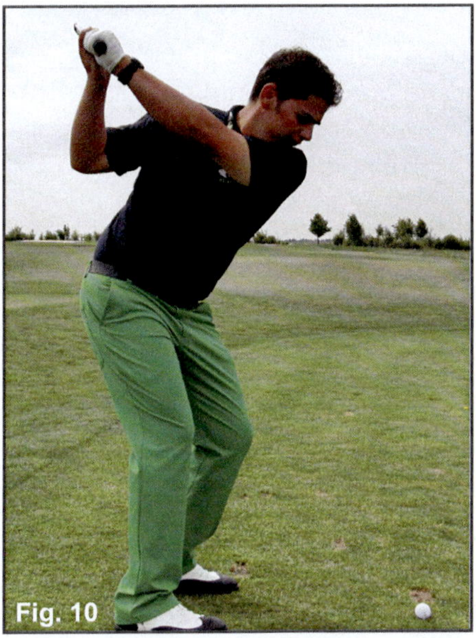
Fig. 10

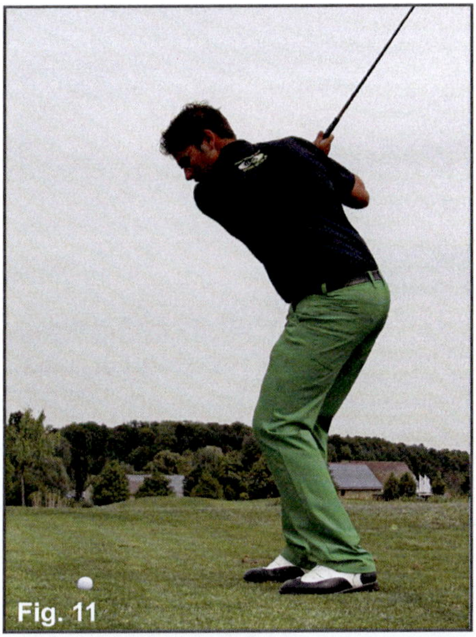
Fig. 11

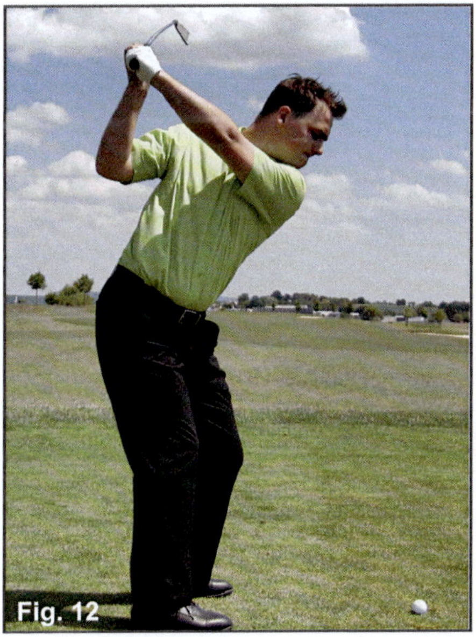
Fig. 12

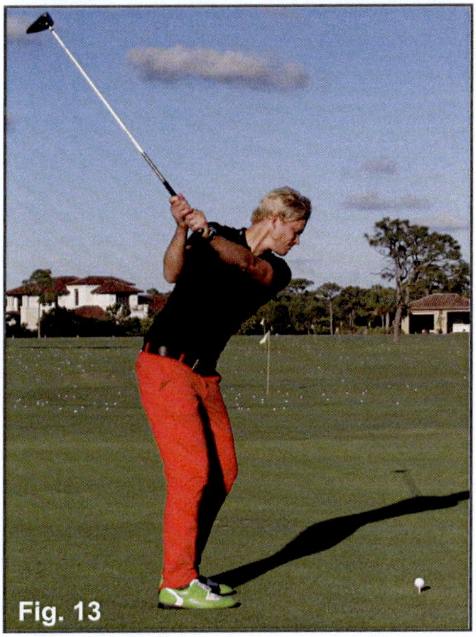
Fig. 13

Downswing

- The downswing is exclusively initiated through the right big toe (see page 88, Fig. 1)
- In doing so, this big toe triggers the rotational push
- The declared goal here is to accelerate **the pelvis** by 67.5 degrees from the-45-degree position (can also be referred to as "zero degrees") in which the ball impact shall take place (see Sketch 1)
- The overall **pelvic rotation** occurs without any motional interruption until the swing finish, parallel to the "target horizon"; altogether, there is a rotation of 135 degrees from the "0 angle" (see Sketch 1)
- The right knee remains next to the "body" (see page 88-89)

SKETCH 1
PELVIC ROTATION

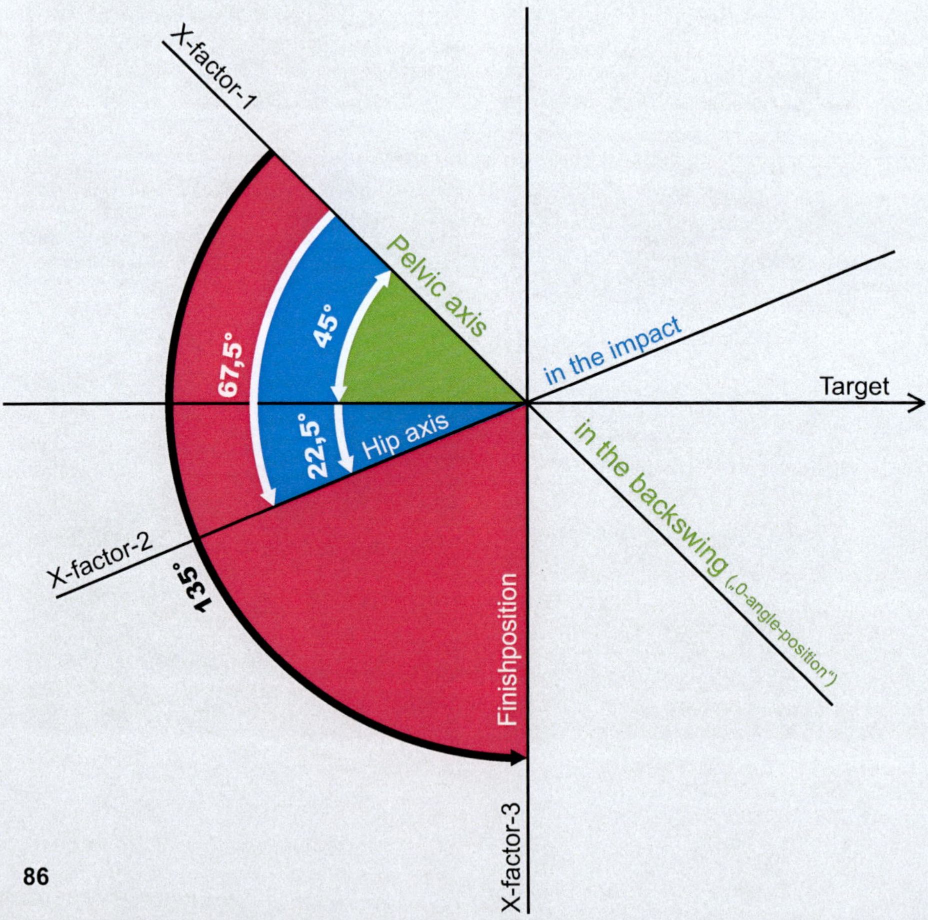

SKETCH 2

SHOULDER ROTATION

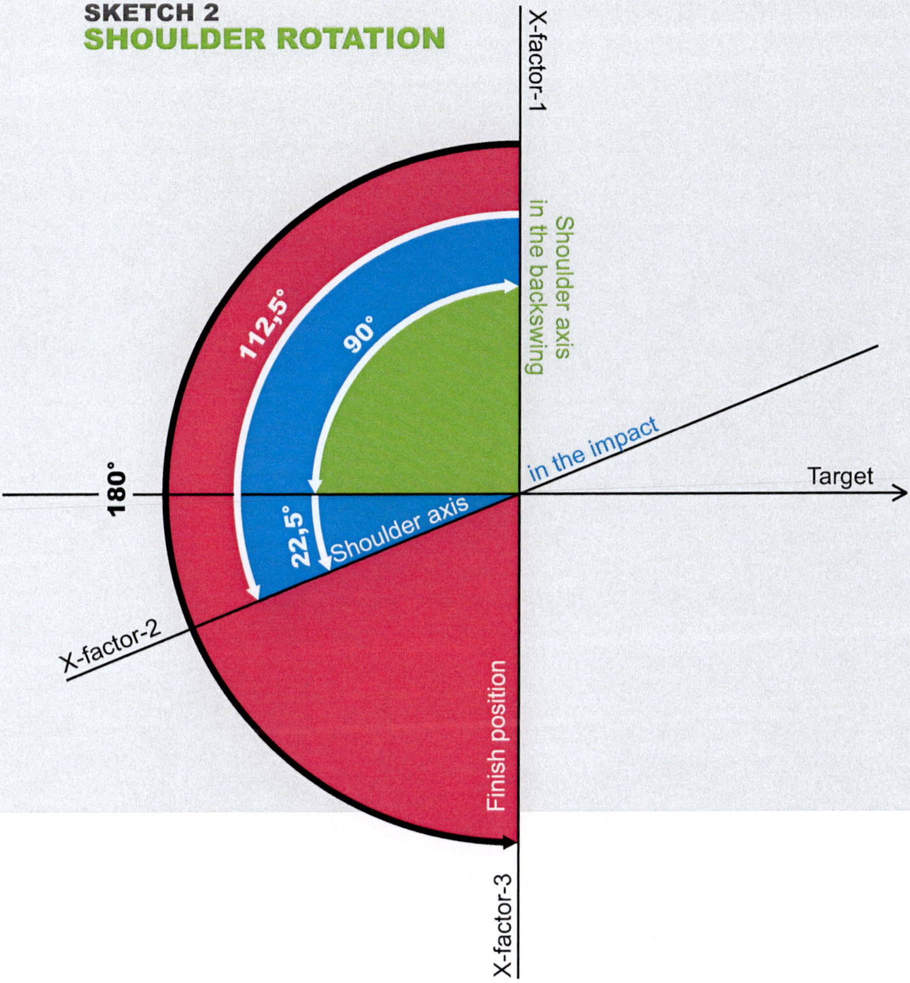

- **The shoulder** rotates in the downswing until ball impact by (90 plus 22.5 degrees) 112.5 degrees (see Sketch 2)
- In doing so, the body's center of gravity is kept stable
- The ball-club head angle is ideally at 0 degrees, or the angle of attack can also be referred to as 90 degrees (see p. 88-89)
- The left upper arm and the chest form a combined unit
- The tempo of the shoulder-arm rotation is faster than that of the legwork
- Both rotations intersect at the moment of impact (see p.89, Fig. 10)
- The centripetal force accelerates the left wrist shortly before the moment of impact. (see p. 88, Fig. 9)

Downswing sequences

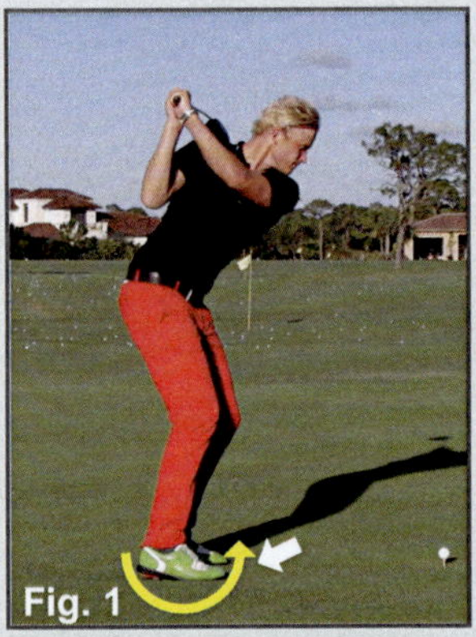
Fig. 1

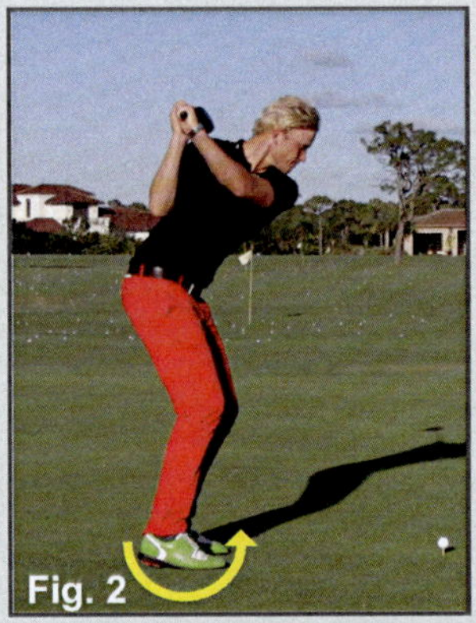
Fig. 2

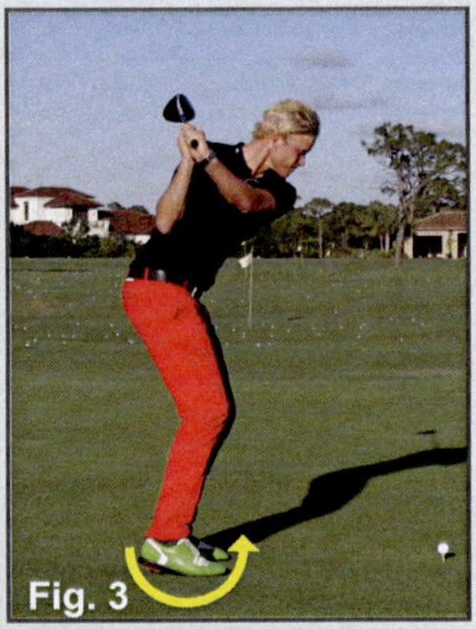
Fig. 3

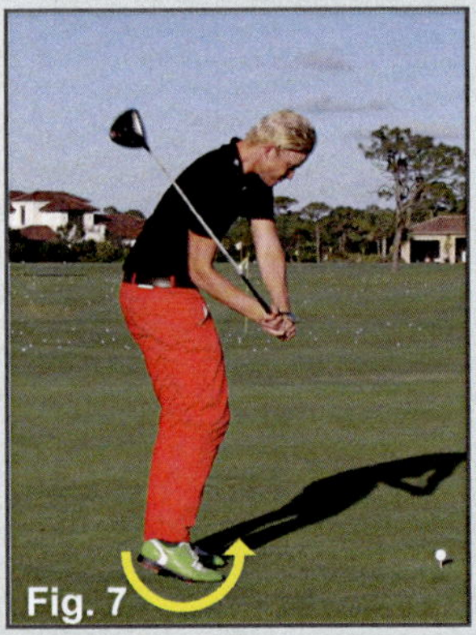
Fig. 7

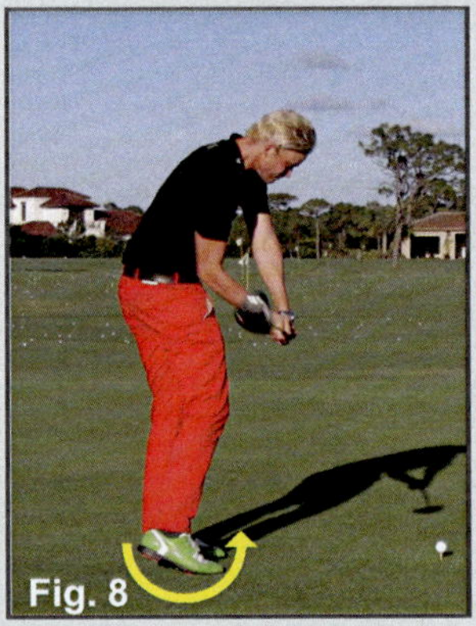
Fig. 8

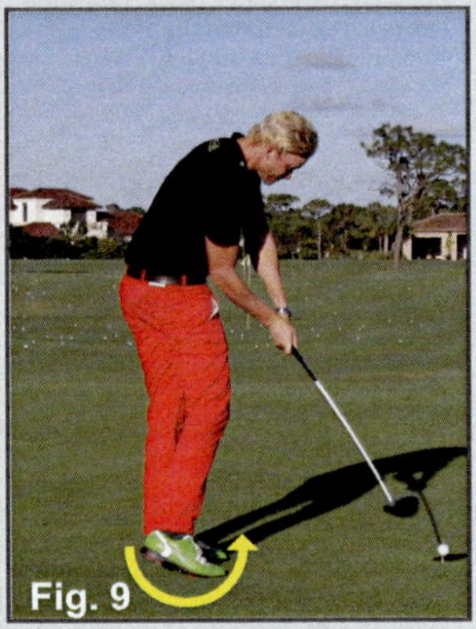
Fig. 9

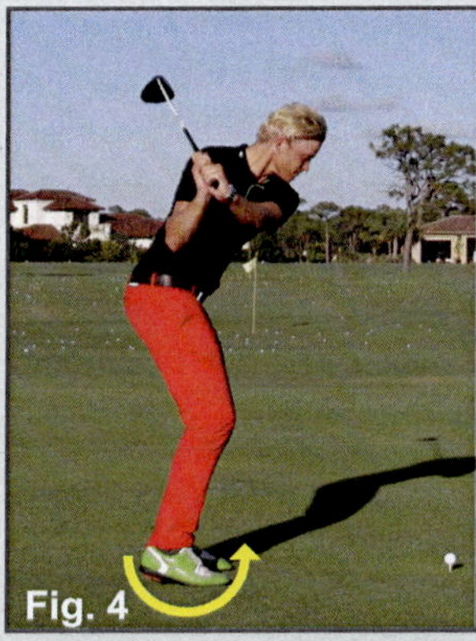

Fig. 4

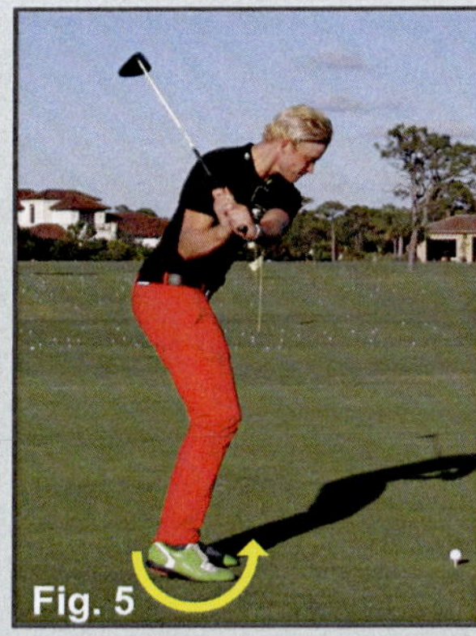

Fig. 5

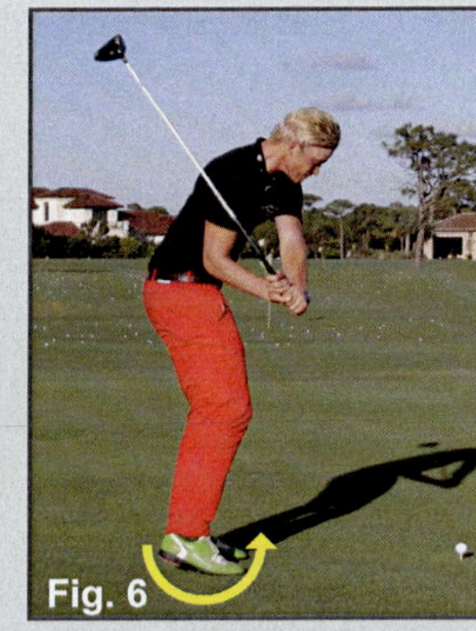

Fig. 6

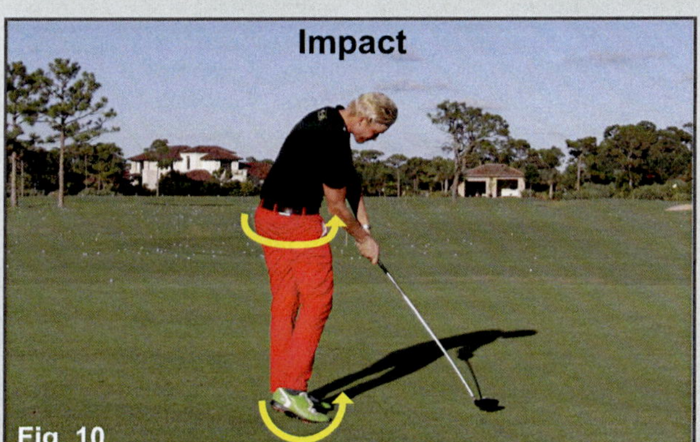

Fig. 10

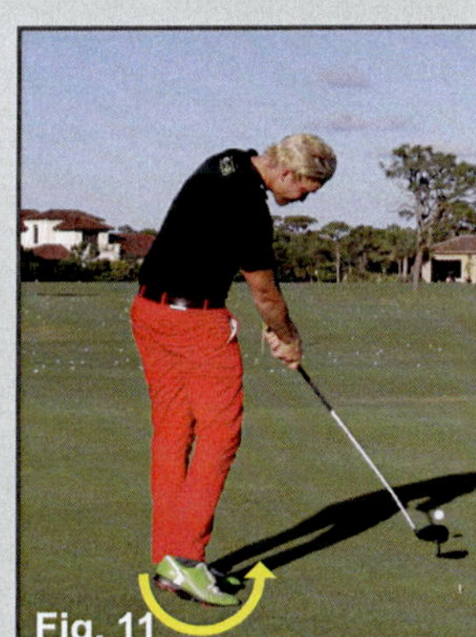

Fig. 11

Perfect X-factor-2
Hip accelerated by 67.5° towards the target, active legwork.

5.3. Difference between active and passive method

PASSIVE METHOD

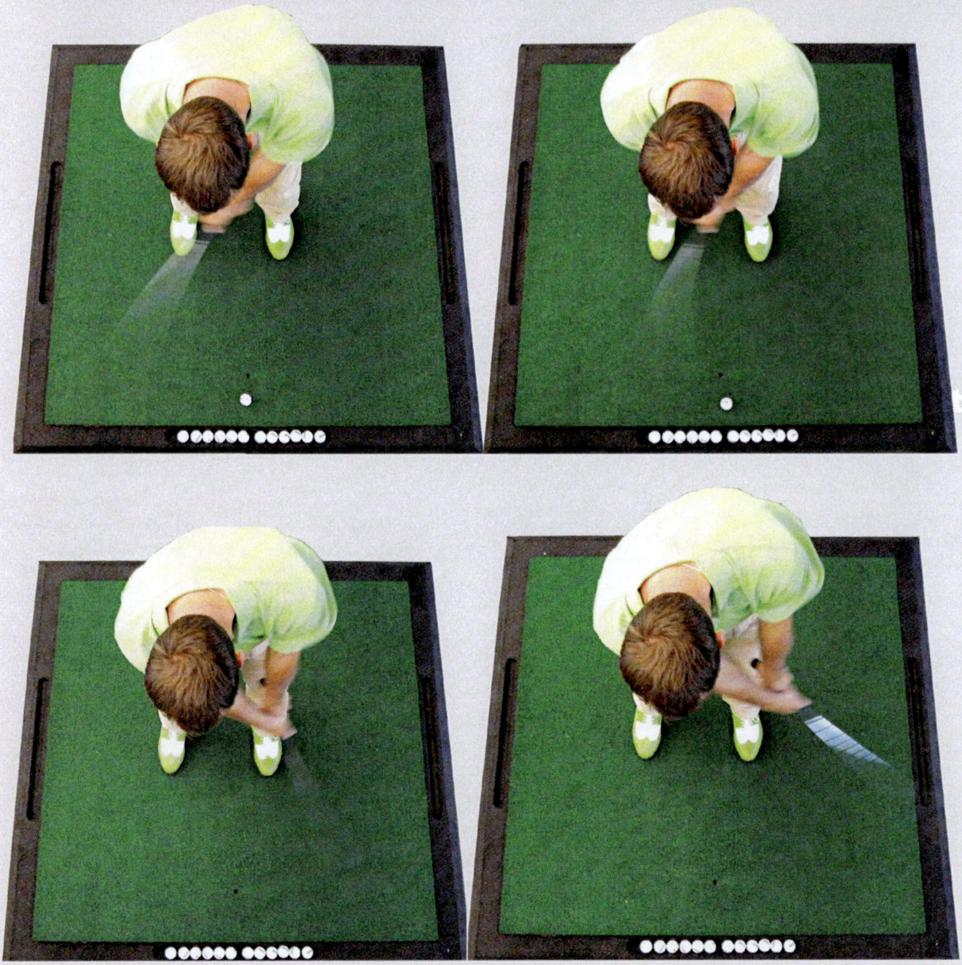

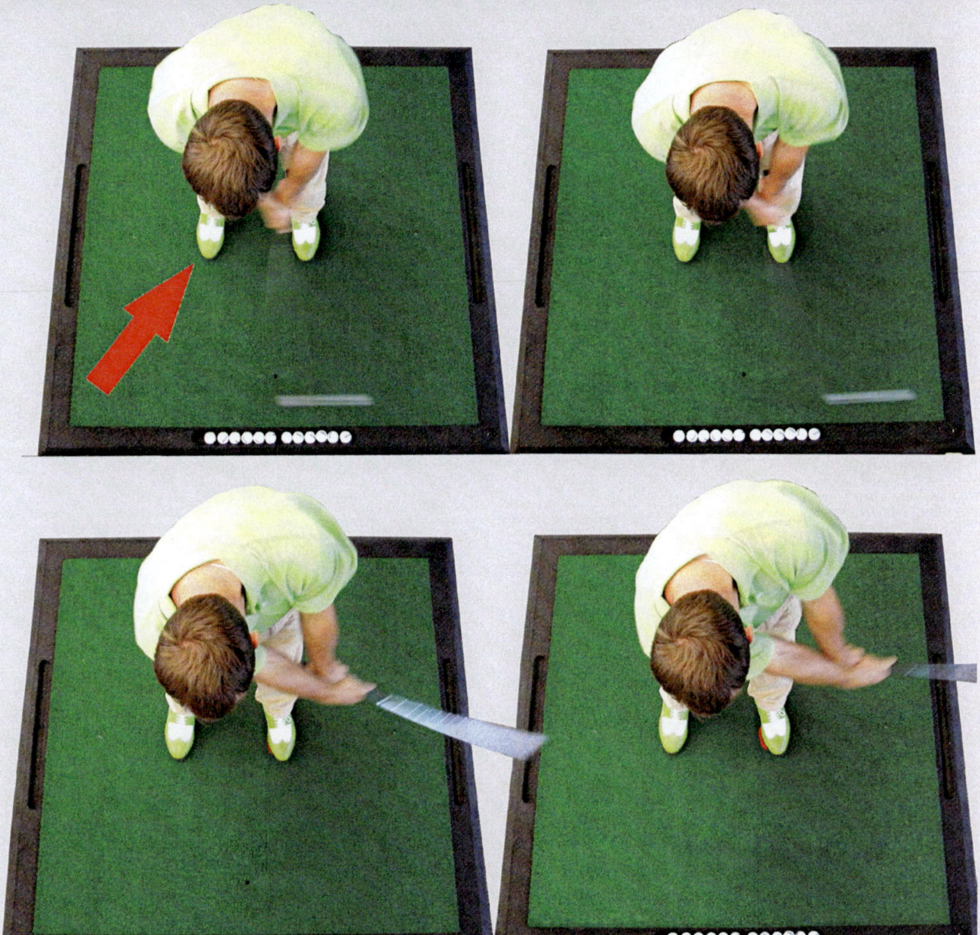

ACTIVE METHOD SIDE VIEW

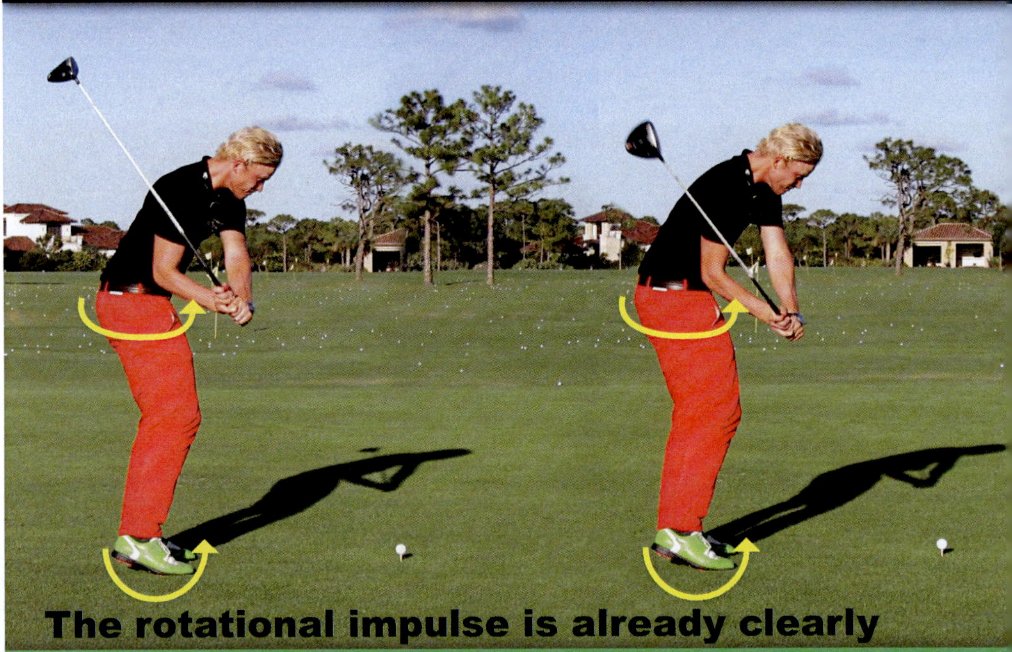
The rotational impulse is already clearly

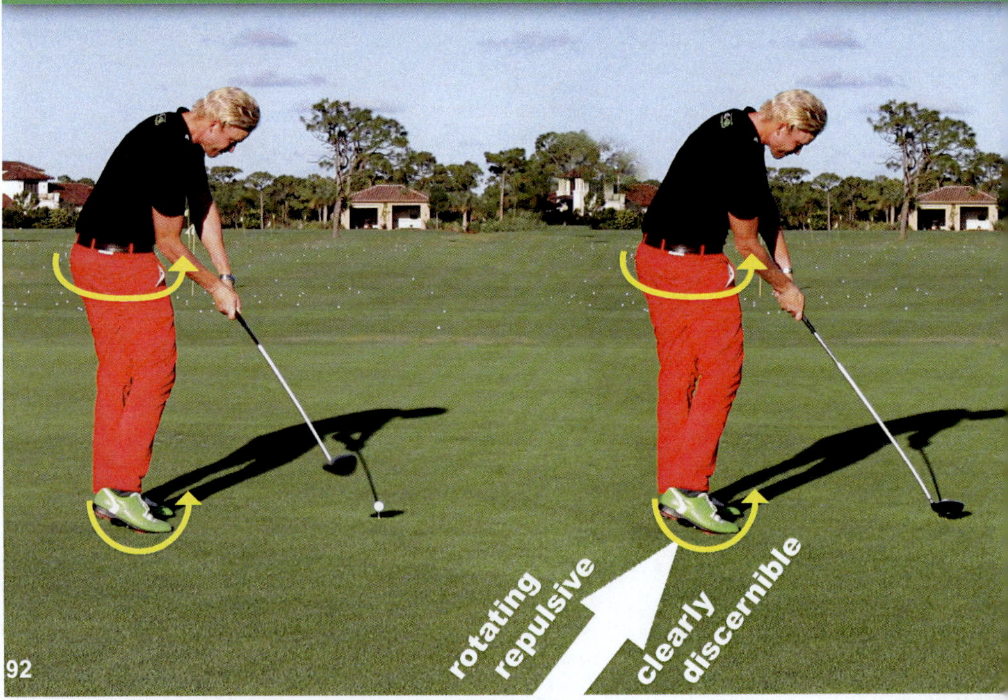
rotating
repulsive
clearly
discernible

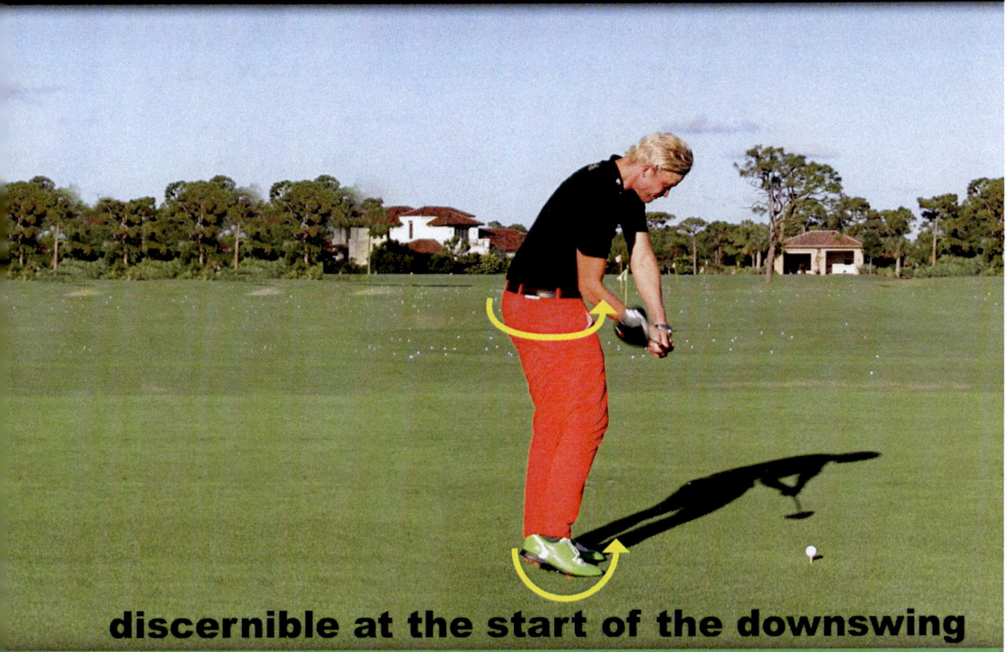

discernible at the start of the downswing

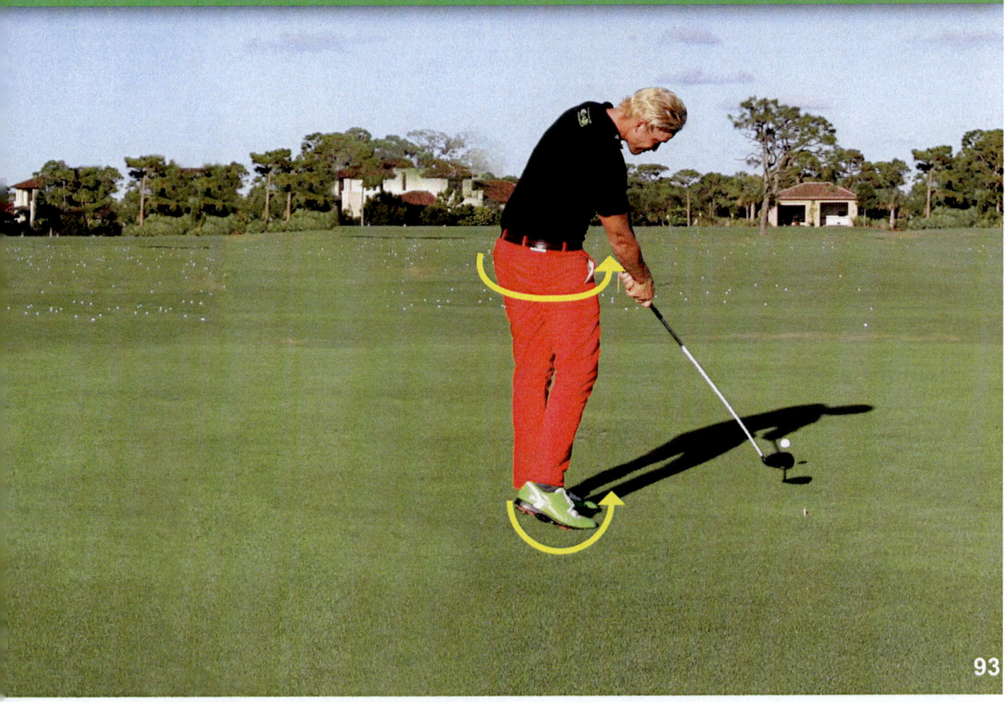

ACTIVE METHOD FRONTAL VIEW

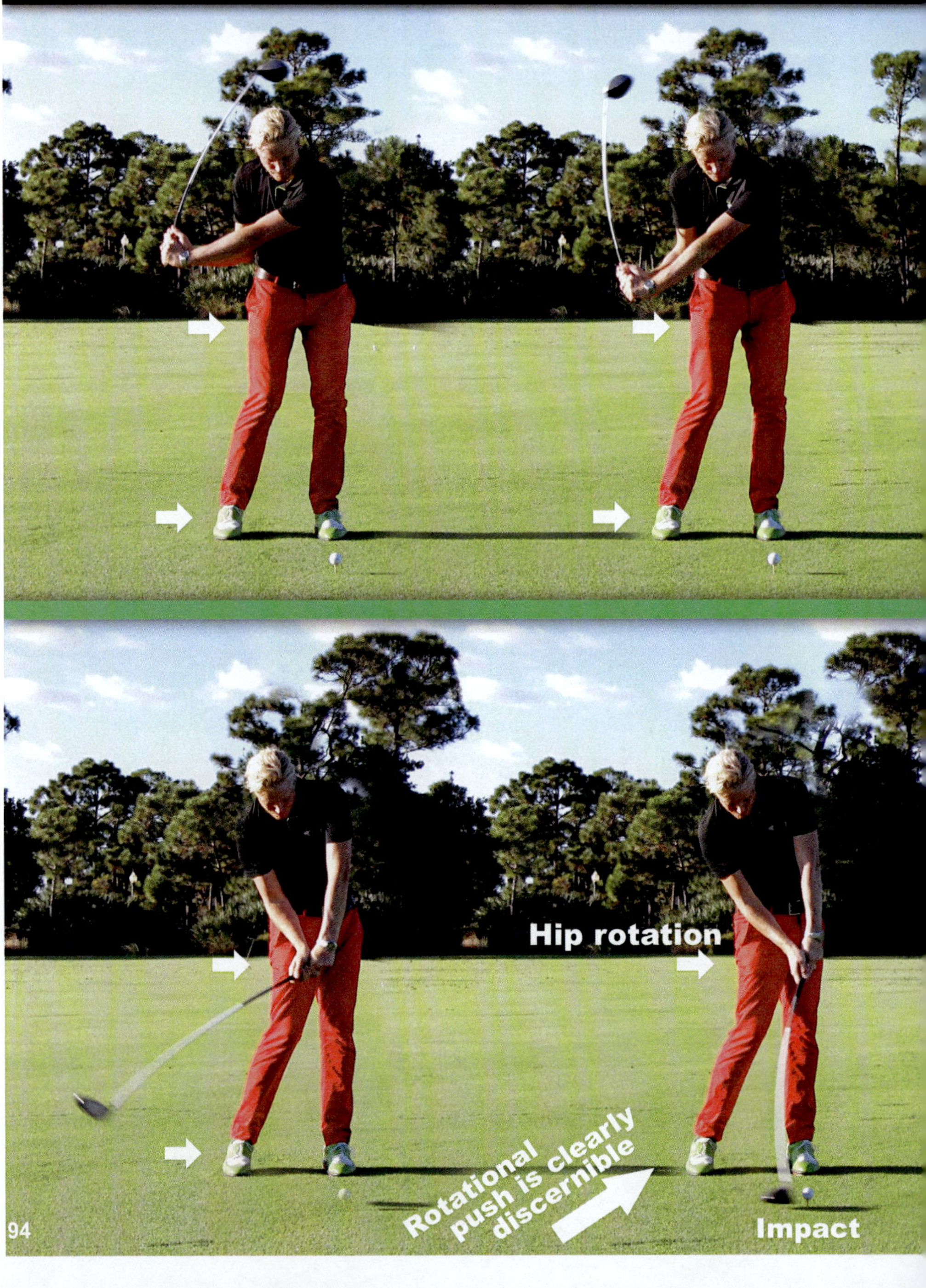

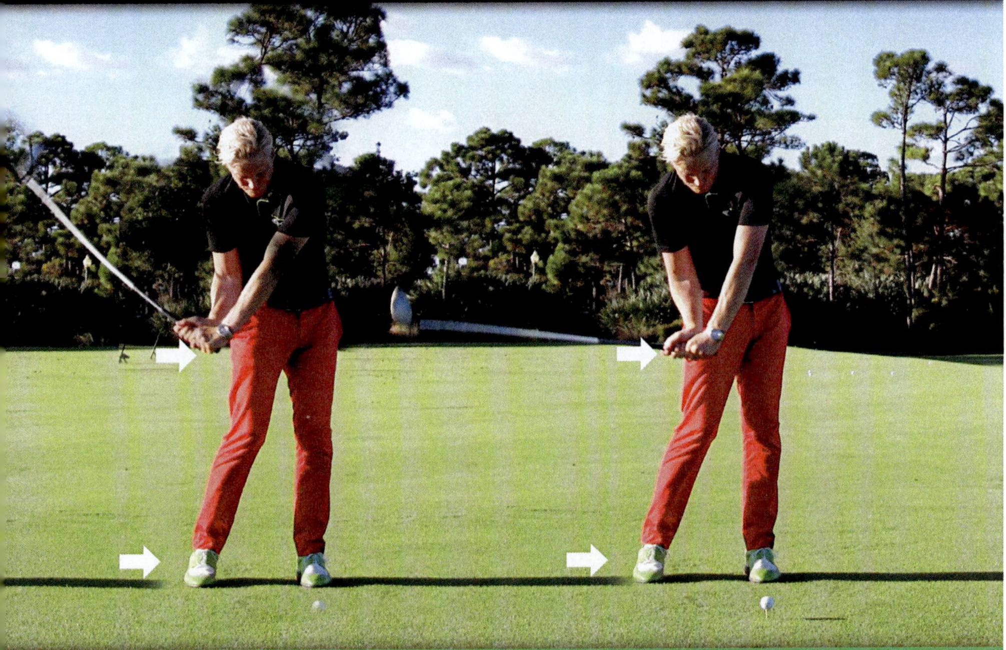

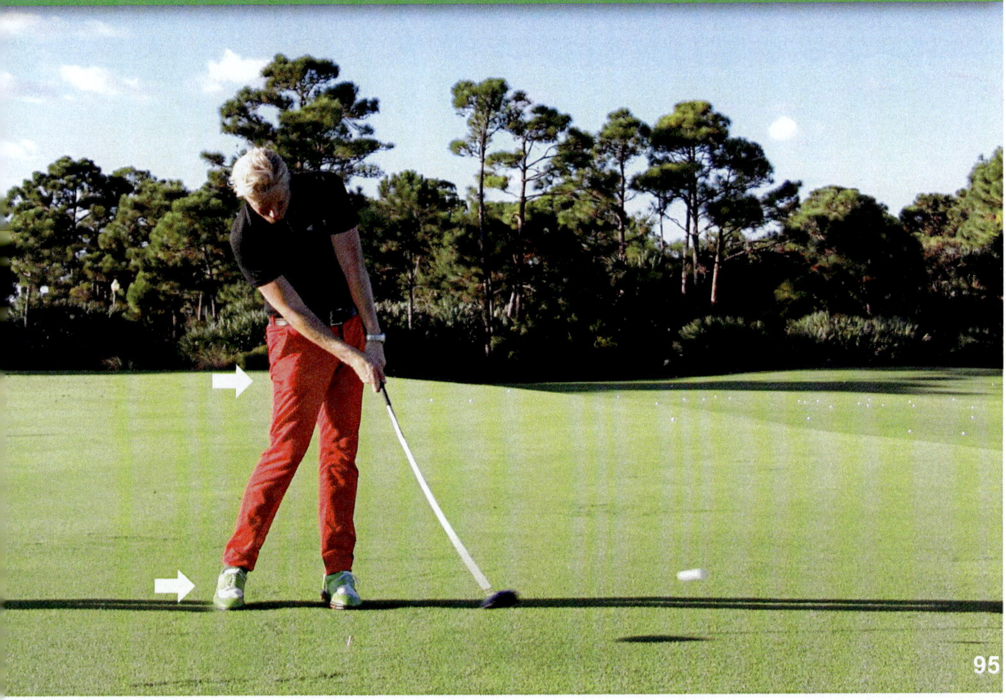

5.3.a. Why is the replacement of passive swing sequences through active swing sequences so important?

With the swing method according to Ben Hogan, one of the main functions of the overall motion sequence is the shifting of body weight to the back leg on the backswing.

The main function of this weight shift is not – as frequently assumed – to generate additional energy for the downswing, but serves to functionally relieve the burden of the knee joint in the leg closest to the target.

Without this shift of weight it would not be possible for the thigh to turn over the knee joint functionally together with the upper body in the downswing and finish.

Because the anatomy of the knee joint does not allow a lateral rotation of the thigh towards the lower leg (the foot area is 'fixed' through ground contact) under the full load of body weight, the body rotation after ball impact can only be carried out if the burden on the knee joint is relieved.

Otherwise evasive (compensatory) modifications are necessary in order to still be able to control the swing phases after ball impact.

In the most frequently found execution of this evasive movement, the golfer stands on the heel of the front foot (backward lean, imbalance) and turns over the heel of the shoe on the downswing.

The reverse possibility, to turn

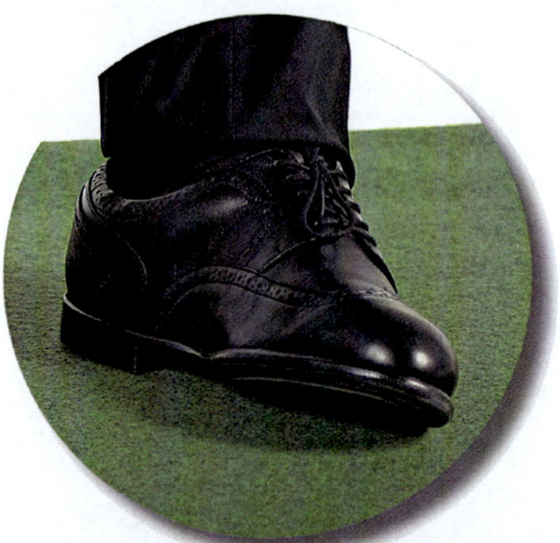

Examples of clear backward lean ➡ imbalance

over the toe area of the front foot (forward lean, imbalance), is observed more seldom.

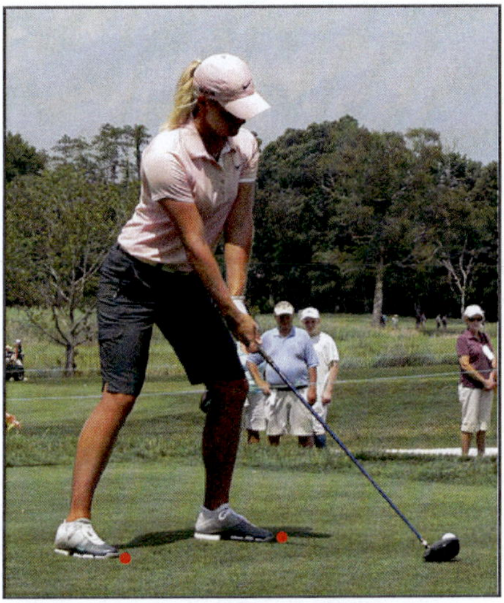

Suzann Pettersen shows us an example of this. She had to recover from a chronic hip injury in 2010.

The causes for this can only be treated through the Turning Shoe plus the Golf-Active-Method FREE-RELEASE®.

However, imbalances entail the great disadvantage that the golfer no longer swings in body balance, but in a more pronounced backward or forward lean. But this is also physiologically very detrimental to performance.

We also discover a loss of energy transfer values to the golf ball.

Imbalance in the swing always signifies a loss of swing energy and diminished precision.

There is also the fact that the evasive motion of the forward or backward lean together with the right-left shifting of weight creates a hypermobile center of gravity for the body.

As a result, the body's center of gravity is moved and accelerated in all three spatial coordinates during the swing.

A controlled, guided swing is hardly possible where the body's center of gravity is so unstable.

The shifting of body weight (approx. 85%) to the backswing foot employed with the swing method according to Ben Hogan has another crucial disadvantage: under such a strong weight load the muscles in the backswing leg will be blocked, whereby active legwork with dynamic hip acceleration on the downswing cannot be executed.

The sports channel ESPN, in cooperation with Greg Rose and John Brenkus, confirmed this static situation. In the course of measurements with Rory McIlroy, Rose determined that on the downswing he accelerates his pelvis with the help of diagonal abdominal muscles, i.e. he "tears" the pelvis (with 720 degrees/sec.) forward twice as fast as all other golfers.

In this swing method the arm/shoulder rotation on the downswing is almost always "too fast". With the "Golf Balance Trainer" (GBT) I have developed – a special mechanical exercise device for motion training of legwork during the golf swing – it can be very clearly proven that the shifting of weight to the backswing foot makes active legwork impossible.

You will find motion videos about GBT at :
www.golf-balance-trainer.com

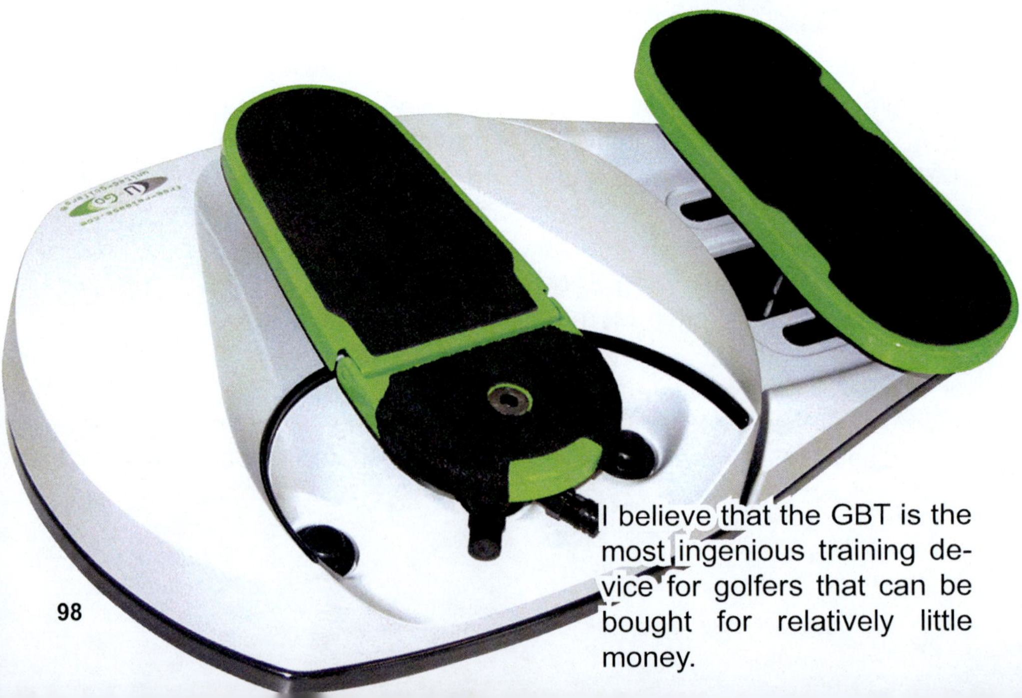

I believe that the GBT is the most ingenious training device for golfers that can be bought for relatively little money.

Training for active legwork

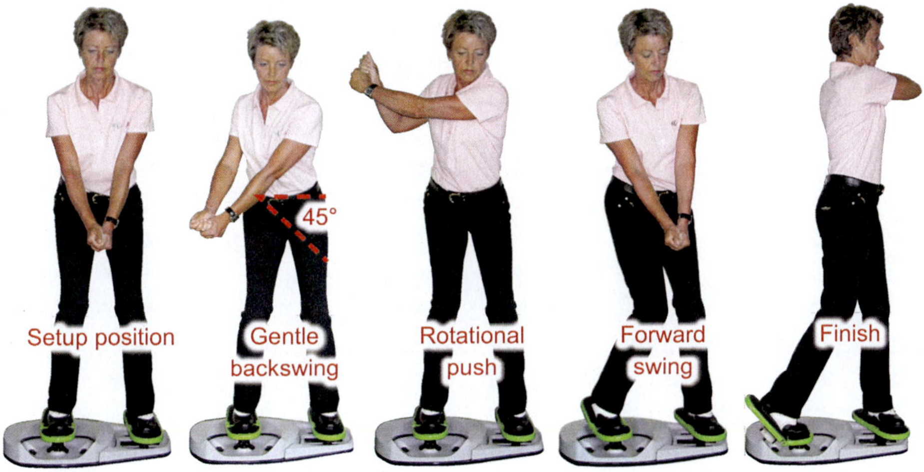

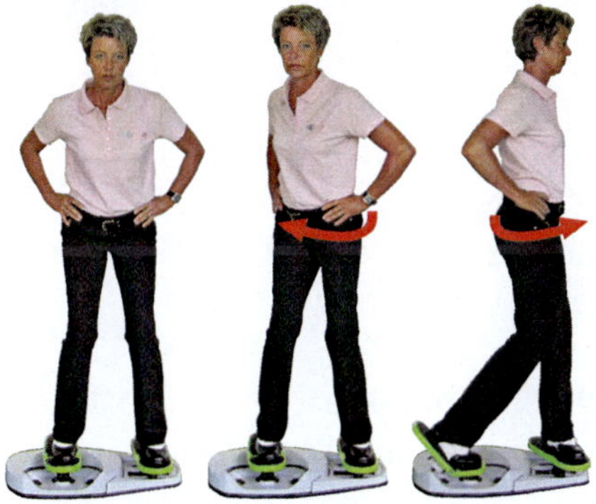

■ Conditioning the motion sequence
■ Strengthening the leg muscles
■ Feeling & finding balance
■ Stabilization of rotational push

- Hands on the hips
- Gentle backswing
- Launch the backswing foot towards the end position via the big toe

■ Strengthening the arm and shoulder muscles

- Take the Thera-Band® in both hands, under tension
- Secure arms on the hips
- Gentle backswing
- During the backswing, pull the Thera-Band® lengthwise with the hand on the backswing side
- Actively launch the backswing foot forward via the big toe
- During the downswing, pull the Thera-Band® lengthwise with the hand on the downswing side

Theraband

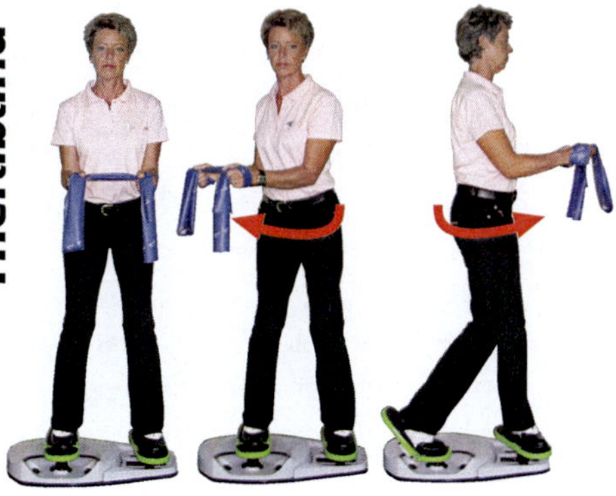

View beyond the horizon: carving ski technique

This form of energetically and physiologically inefficient functional relief of the knee joint by means of accelerating the body's center of gravity may be well known to all those who were active in alpine skiing before the introduction of the carving ski: The "high-low leg turning" motional sequence practiced according to the control technique at that time fulfilled the same function as the shifting of weight in the swing method according to Ben Hogan.

In the description of methodology for ski instruction at that time, the motional function of "high-low leg turning" was described as follows: "The goal is functional relief of the knee joint so that the thigh can turn over the knee joint until the end position of the joint is reached and the lower leg is also brought into a position to make a change of direction."

Although the "high-low leg turning" motional sequence was in accordance with the skiing control technique at that time, this method caused dangerous and structurally harmful torsion loads in the knee joint.

But also with regard to performance, the control technique at that time – just like the Ben Hogan method – was far from optimal, because with the "high-low leg turning" technique the curve cannot be ridden on an exact line, but only in a larger radius.

Severe losses of time in the downhill run were the result of this curve skiing technique. When the carving technique was introduced it very quickly became clear that this method was much more efficient and healthier than the previous control technique.

Interestingly enough, in biomechanical terms the carving technique is very similar to the GAM FREE-RELEASE®, because with both new methods it is possible to fix the body's hypermobile center of gravity according to the old method.

And as with the carving technique, the improvements with the GAM

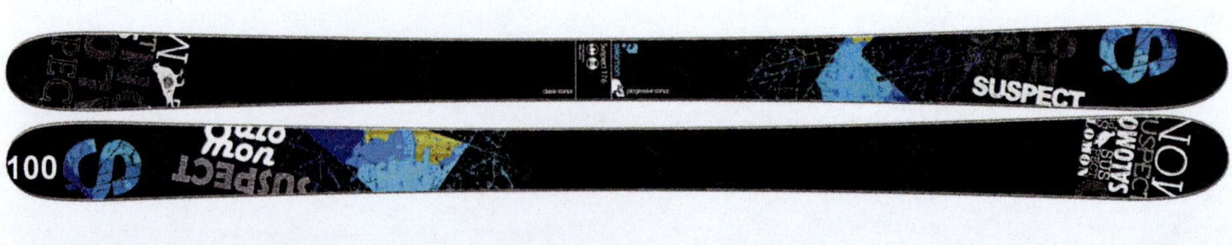

FREE-RELEASE® method can also be verified very easily through measurements. It is common knowledge that the carving technique has become completely accepted in terms of method as well as hardware in the sphere of recreational and competitive skiing.

The shifting of weight in the backswing implemented with the Ben Hogan method blocks any controllable and active legwork. A static state that can only be overcome by means of an auxiliary motion – the lateral shifting of the hip towards the target – is created through the shifting of weight onto the back leg.

Ask a physicist whether it is better from an energetic viewpoint in order to achieve a highest possible rotational speed (club head), to first thrust a body and then turn or to rotate around a stable axis. Every physics professor will immediately confirm that the GAM FREE-RELEASE® is much more energetically efficient than the swing model according to Ben Hogan.

A crucial disadvantage of the auxiliary motion of shifting the hip with the swing method according to Ben Hogan is that the body's center of gravity is hypermobile.

In turn, the body's hypermobile center of gravity means that the quality of ball impact is no longer controllable and repeatable.

The proof of this is provided by measurements of the ball impact angle using a Doppler radar device, but also the "PGATour.com" statistics for target precision (driving accuracy).

Any mathematics teacher will agree with me: if every second ball does not land on the fairway (Phil Mickelson driving accuracy: 52%), then in mathematical terms we speak of a result coincidence.

The described shifting of weight to the backswing foot with the swing model from Ben Hogan also has a serious biomechanical weakness: Due to the unequally higher weight load of the backswing leg, the muscle groups there cannot start early enough with the active legwork, which is why the hip is not

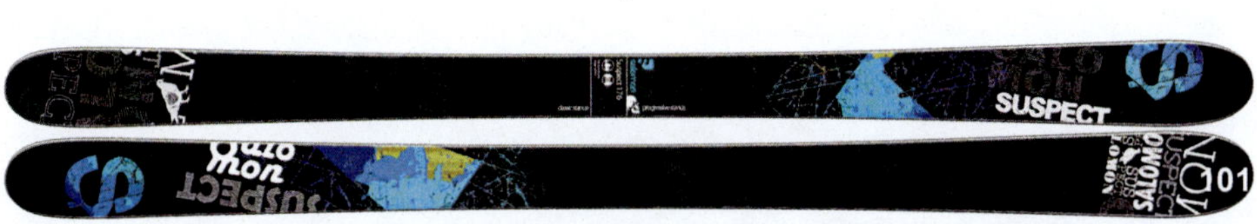

sufficiently accelerated towards the target in the downswing. Shifting of weight in the backswing leads to time-delayed, asynchronous legwork in the downswing.

I refer to this position – which is extremely disadvantageous for the development of higher club head velocity – as a biomechanically passive state: the legwork with the rotational push can only be activated after the hip is positioned clearly towards the target (laterally) on the downswing. But since this motional sequence clearly employs the legwork too late (asynchronous), it is no longer possible to reach the optimal rotational acceleration of the hips on the downswing.

In sum, the passive legwork with the swing model developed by Ben Hogan has the following disadvantages:

1. In contrast to the GAM FREE-RELEASE®, the generation and transfer of swing energy does not occur by employing the powerful muscle groups of the legs plus the gluteus muscles.

2. X-factor 2 (identifying the angle of the hips/shoulders at the moment of impact) is either zero or – where the hips are slightly rotated – the rotation is performed in anticipation so that it does not contribute energetically. Anticipation means that the rotation of the hips is not active and controlled, but, rather an anticipatory movement.

Result: Energetic disadvantages and uncontrollable quality of ball impact.

3. In contrast to GAM FREE-RELEASE®, the body's center of gravity is not fixed, but hypermobile. The path covered by the navel (or another fixed point on the body) in this connection is the optical indicator for shifting the body's center of gravity in the course of the swing.

Due to the instability of the body's center of gravity, precise swing management and control is virtually impossible and the impact quality depends on coincidence.

Now you can surely understand in more detail, which is why the GAM FREE-RELEASE® provides the golfer with crucial competitive advantages.

Thanks to today's widespread Doppler radar measuring instruments the GAM FREE-RELEASE® performance advantage can also be objectified very easily.

We were able to measure a peak performance improvement of up to 35% among amateurs. The average performance improvement is 16%.

We were able to measure peak performance improvement (Smash7) of up to 18% among Tour players. The average in this group is 12%.

This is potential for improvement, which nobody – whether pro or amateur – can forego in the future if they do not want to fall behind in their athletic competitive ability.

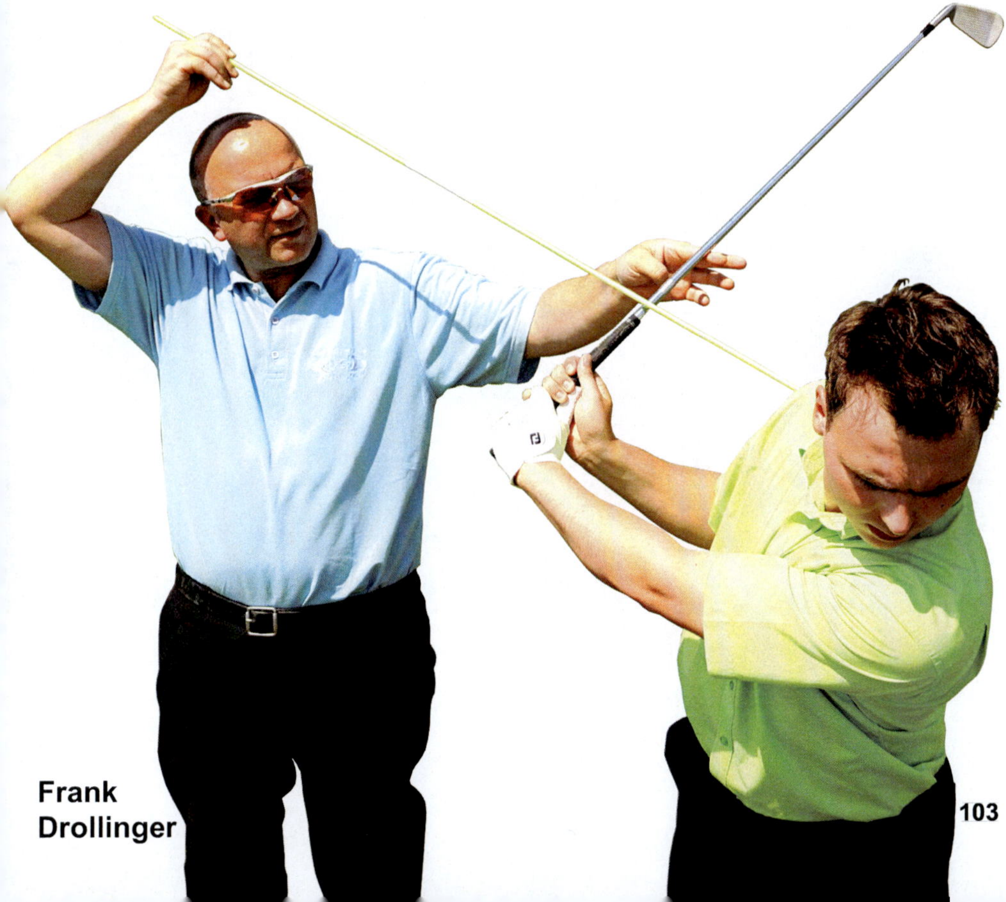

Example of passive legwork: shoulder, hip, leg & foot

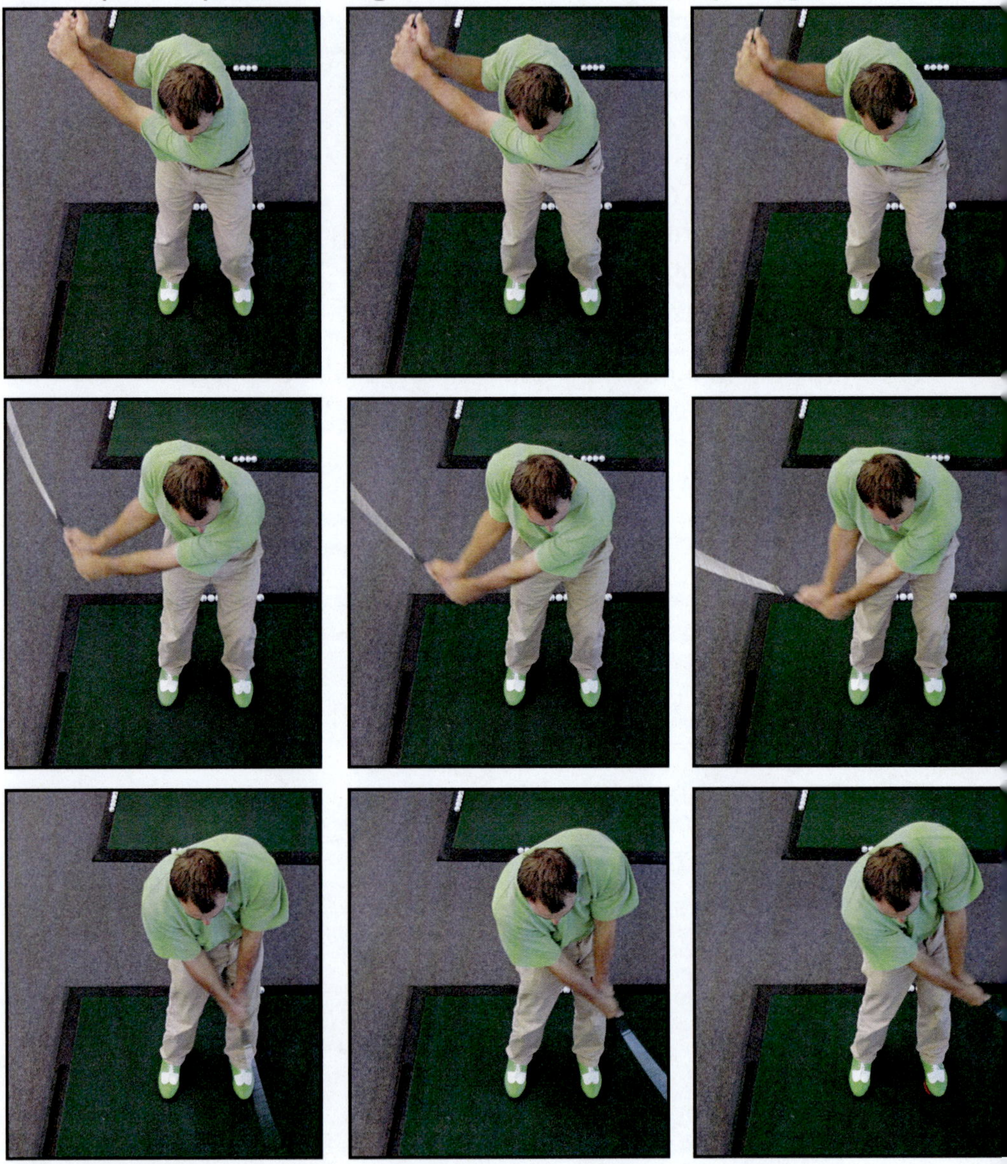

Even after the moment of impact the right heel is still on the ground, a sign o passive legwork.

rotation is "followed" by the arms

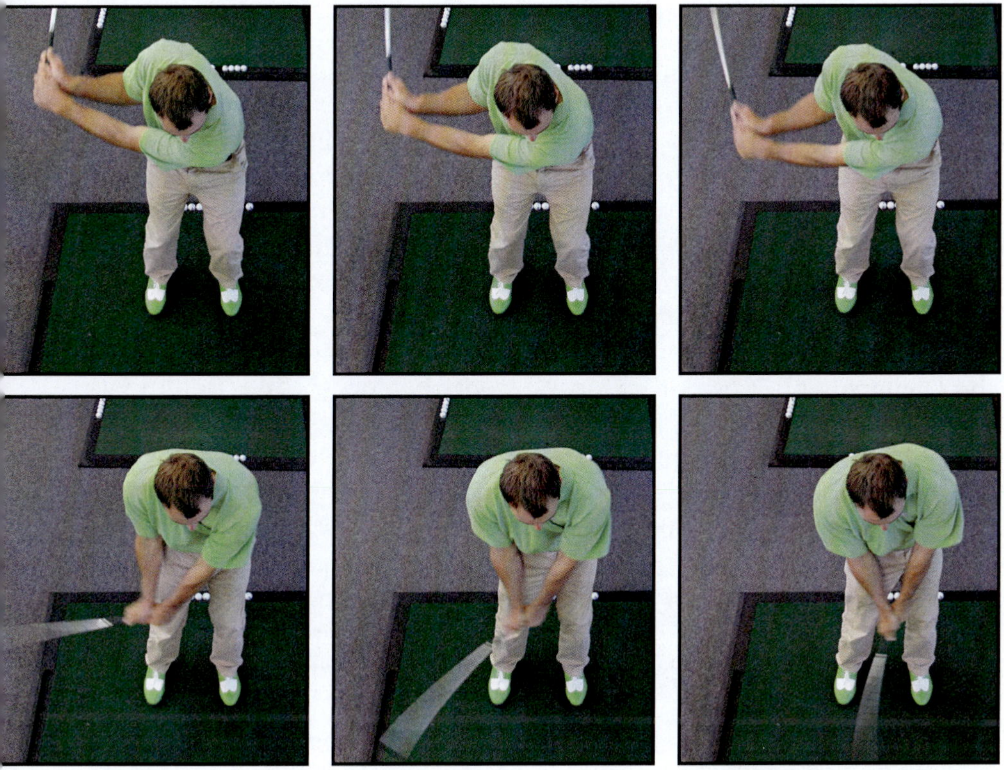

X-factor-2
There is no energetic effect because of passive legwork

Passive legwork:

- **Non-physiological**
- **Outdated kinematics**
- **Lacking rotational push**
- **Reduced energy transfer**
- **Deficient ball impact quality**

The question I asked a talented individual in May 2010: "Who worked with you the past 10 years in athletic & swing training and taught you this passive motion?" After my instruction he had the European Tour card at the end of the year (December 2010)!

5.3.b. Why is the Golf-Active-Method FREE-RELEASE® the world's healthiest method?

I have created a natural motion which is consistent with human structure after starting with an unnatural motion which works against the physical laws of human anatomy.

The University of Tübingen determined in the course of a broadly based kinematic study that during a "textbook" golf swing that is performed according to the Ben Hogan method, forces of approx. **14 Nm** per kg of the player's body weight in the form of torsional and shearing force loads affect the body, particularly the lumbar spinal region and the 'load chain' comprised of the hip joint, knee joint and ankle joint.

In a Tour player these load effects – based on 300 playing or training days with 200 swings each over the course of a year – add up to the almost unbelievable figure of **75,600,000 Nm**!

If you realize with the aid of these figures which substantial burdens have a lasting harmful effect on the musculoskeletal system of a golf player, from a sports medicine viewpoint it is only logical that all Tour players suffer injuries.

It is logical that during a tournament day up to 144 treatments will be administered by the pros in the physiotherapy bus. It is also understandable why taking painkillers (such as diclofenac) is harmful to the kidneys and has become an almost daily prerequisite for being able to play at all in the realm of professional golf.

The entire sports medicine complex pertaining to the topic "stress impairment and stress reduction with golf swing" fills a three-day seminar in my advanced training program for physicians, orthopedists and sports medicine specialists. That is why the health-related aspects and advantages of GAM FREE-RELEASE® in comparison with conventional swing techniques can only be presented in bullet points at this juncture.

The GAM FREE-RELEASE® – in the hardware combination with the Turning Shoe – is the healthiest golf swing method of all.

The Turning Shoe with its "turning sole mechanical system" in the swing phase after the moment of impact reduces the harmful burdens on the body, particularly the joints. Measurements were performed or exact quantification of stress reduction at the University of Tübingen Institute of Sports Science. In doing so, it was determined that the Turning Shoe reduces the effects of forces harmful to the joints by up to 99%.

The GOLF-MEDICAL-COACHES trained in our advanced training program for sports medicine specialists can provide competent advice about the preventive and therapeutic use of the Turning Shoe and the FREE-RELEASE-Method®.

The optimizations of the new GAM FREE-RELEASE® turn an unhealthy motion into a healthy motion.

Disadvantages of Ben Hogan method:

- The lateral and simultaneously rotational shifting of weight in the backswing acts like "P80-grit sandpaper" on the articular cartilage of the ankle, knee and hip joints.
- The articular cartilage will be damaged with every swing. This is not so with Golf-Active-Method FREE-RELEASE®.
- The diagonal torsional load on the spine leads to one-sided wear and tear of the articular cartilage and intervertebral discs so that painful inflammations arise here, as with Annika Sörenstam or Tiger Woods.
- **The passive legwork is responsible for the very substantial strain affecting the pelvis and lumbar vertebrae. For instance, a player such as Jesper Parnevik has broken the L5 lumbar**

vertebrae three times, and 97 artificial hip joints (left and right) were implanted.

- But the torsional resistances in the hip, knee and ankle joints as well as the shinbone are so severe that fatigue fractures, osteoarthritis, cruciate ligament ruptures and chronic supination of the left ankle joint lead to injuries which necessitate artificial hip joints, etc.

Protection for golfing children!

It is especially important to protect golfing children and adolescents. Their articular cartilage does not have any 'voice' which reports to the often very responsible parents. All these burdens and injuries can be prevented with a 99% probability thanks to the GAM FREE-RELEASE® overall system.

The risk of injury is reduced by a factor of 15 with the GAM FREE-RELEASE®.

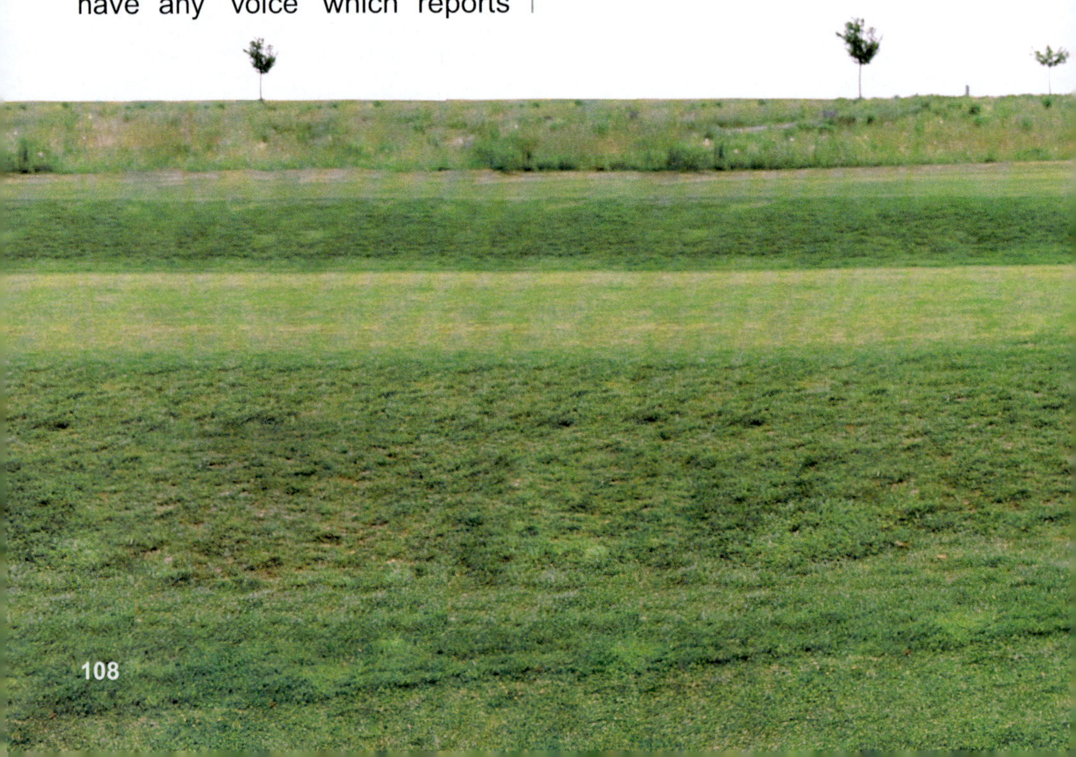

“The Golf-Active-Method FREE-RELEASE® system can absolutely be described as a high-end system and as a control technique.”

Frank Drollinger

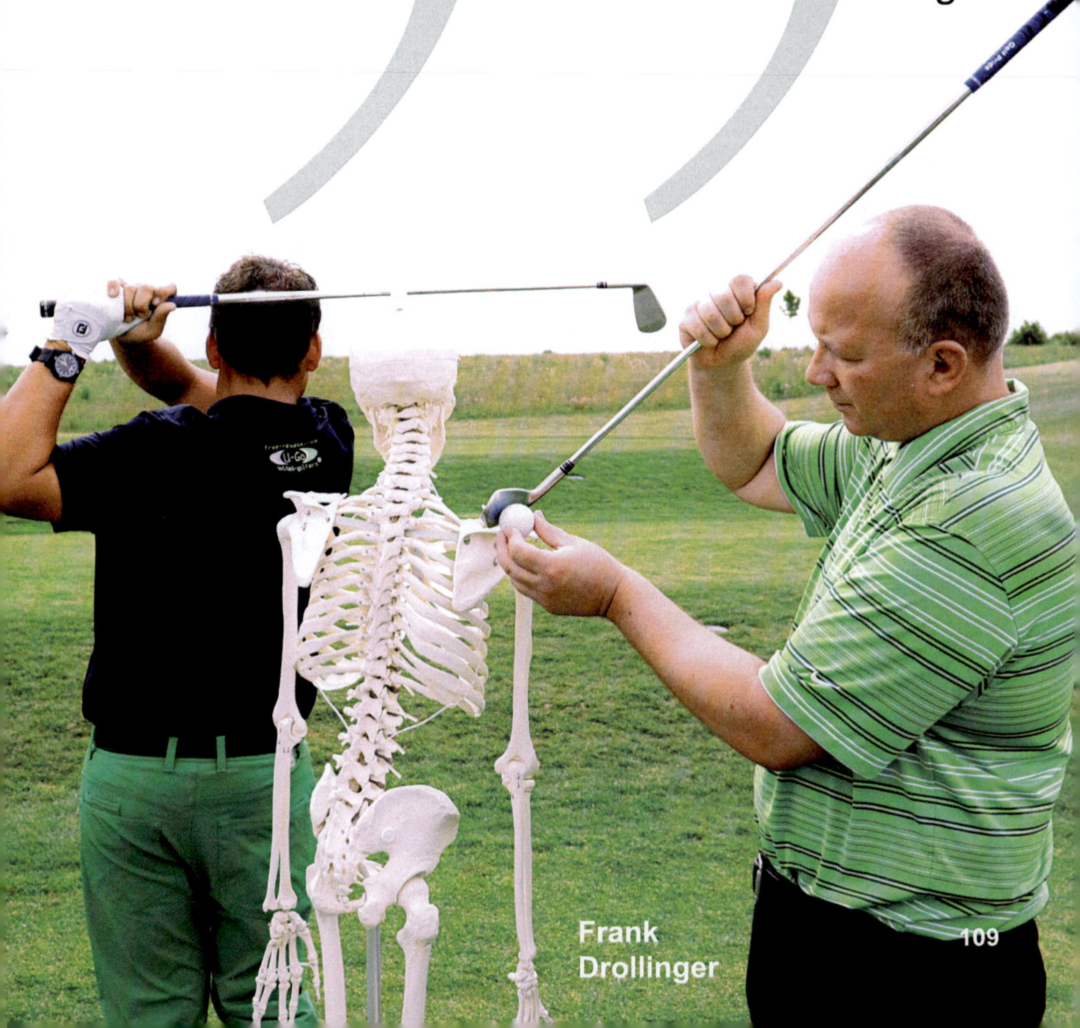

Frank Drollinger

Excursus

Rules experts:
Golf is a gentleman's game. The basic foundations are sportsmanship, fairness and courtesy.

From time to time rules experts claim that the rules do not pay attention to the health of the athletes.

But then I ask myself why drug tests are performed?

For instance, this is also not in the rules!

Does a golfer who has an injury play according to the basic principles of the Rules of Golf?

For instance, what happens if a player is bleeding? Do the (rules officials) referees allow him to walk across the course? Certainly not!

What happens in the event of a leg fracture like Tiger Woods had at the US Open in 2008? He worsened his state of health due to the torsions.

The spirit of the game deals with the behavior of participants and those responsible.

The word "sportsmanship" relates to ethics, or the golfer's moral behavior. According to that, an athlete may not take part in any tournament with an injury.

An athlete may also not burden himself through motion and hardware.

All associations have signed the IOC Charter and pledged in writing to comply with it.

An unequivocal opinion is rendered in Chapter 7 of the Medical Code, which also applies to all golfers since 2009:

"No practice constituting any form of physical injury or physiological should be acceptable."

5.3.c. Alignment

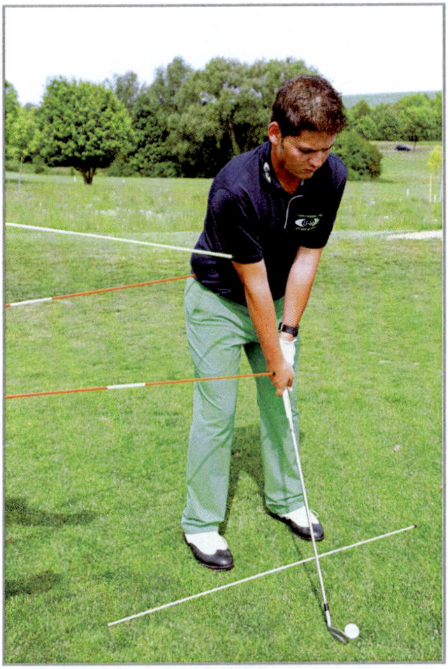

The correct alignment of the body's axes in the setup is an important element of the Golf-Active-Method FREE-RELEASE®.

At this juncture, all of the body's axes are aligned parallel and positioned at an angle of 90 degrees towards the "target horizon".

The foot, knee, hip, shoulder and head axis form one unit in this connection.

"My mission is the introduction of functional, personalized health management in golf. The 'Turning Shoe Zero Stress Health Promoter' and the Golf-Active-Method FREE-RELEASE® play the principal roles here."

Frank Drollinger

5.3.d. Placement of target foot

In a study conducted in 2010, California State (Fullerton) Professor Dr. Scott Lynn determined that the torsional strain in the knee joint of the front leg is hardly reduced through the frequently recommended placement of the target foot.

Hence the torsional strain placed on the knee joint is only reduced by 15% if the foot is placed towards the target.

This minimal relief is by no means enough to effectively protect the structures of the knee joint, but also the ankle and hip joint against typical torsion-related damage on a medium and long-term basis.

According to the Ben Hogan golf swing model, the placement of the target foot also remains an non-physiological and thereby fundamentally unhealthy motion sequence.

But in addition to the very limited physiological-sports medicine benefit, the placement of the foot axis is particularly associated with serious biomechanical disadvantages:

The parallelism and axial unity is disturbed through the lateral angulation of the foot axis, not only there, but also in the knee and hip axis. All axes in the foot, hip and knee are brought out of alignment from their actual ideal position.

The target precision and energy transfer will be substantially diminished as a result.

Another biomechanically undesirable consequence with regard to placement of the target foot is that the pivot point for the body rotation is no longer in middle of the foot (the foot's balance point), but is displaced further backward towards the heel. As a result, the golfer's foot placement has an increasing tendency towards an instable backward lean.

No biomechanically disadvantageous makeshift solution such as placement of the foot towards the target is required with GAM

FREE-RELEASE® in order to effectively protect the joints – particularly the knee joint – against torsional impairments. Effective stress reduction is achieved by GAM FREE-RELEASE® hardware through the use of the Turning Shoe. The torsional loads pertaining to the FREE-RELEASE-Method® would be virtually the same without the use of the Turning Shoe.

Our top players therefore place special emphasis on alignment, which is constantly practiced as an individual ritual during training and consolidation of their swing routine.

"Natural kinematics enables a sustainable and repeatable performance improvement in golf. Every minute of training leads to improvement."

Frank Drollinger

5.3.e. The emotional intelligence of top players and their search for swing balance

Good players have distinct motional intuition – I call this "emotional intelligence" – and seek the balance which is not achievable with the swing model according to Ben Hogan due to biomechanical reasons. The door towards implementation of measurable swing balance is opened for the first time with the GAM FREE-RELEASE®.

Only virtually perfect balance measured with foot pressure point plates enables a repeatable ball impact, since there is a direct connection between good 'Balance1' (swing phase: backswing and downswing to ball impact) and the realization of an ideal ball-clubface impact angle.

At this juncture, only GAM FREE-RELEASE® provides the opportunity to reproducibly implement the best values.

In addition to the intuition for balance, emotional intelligence is also characterized by the ability to perceive the body's inner voice and its feedback during the swing. Physiologically detrimental influences of force and a motion which cause injuries provoke the body of any player to make motional modifications in order to avoid pain through neurological feedback from the amygdalae.

An "emotionally intelligent" player can perceive this process. However, exactly this perception and control process also makes the golf swing according to the Ben Hogan model difficult for a professional golfer to control and unnecessarily complicated.

Particularly at this point the golf swing according to GAM FREE-RELEASE® substantially reduces the motional coordination effort.

Since the golf swing is a motion that is executed to a large extent physiologically torsion-free and stress-free, the golfer does not have to guide the swing against the body's compensatory evasive motions.

“Our body knows exactly what we do to it without the use of “Turning Shoe Zero Stress” and GAM FREE-RELEASE®. It forgets nothing.”

Frank Drollinger

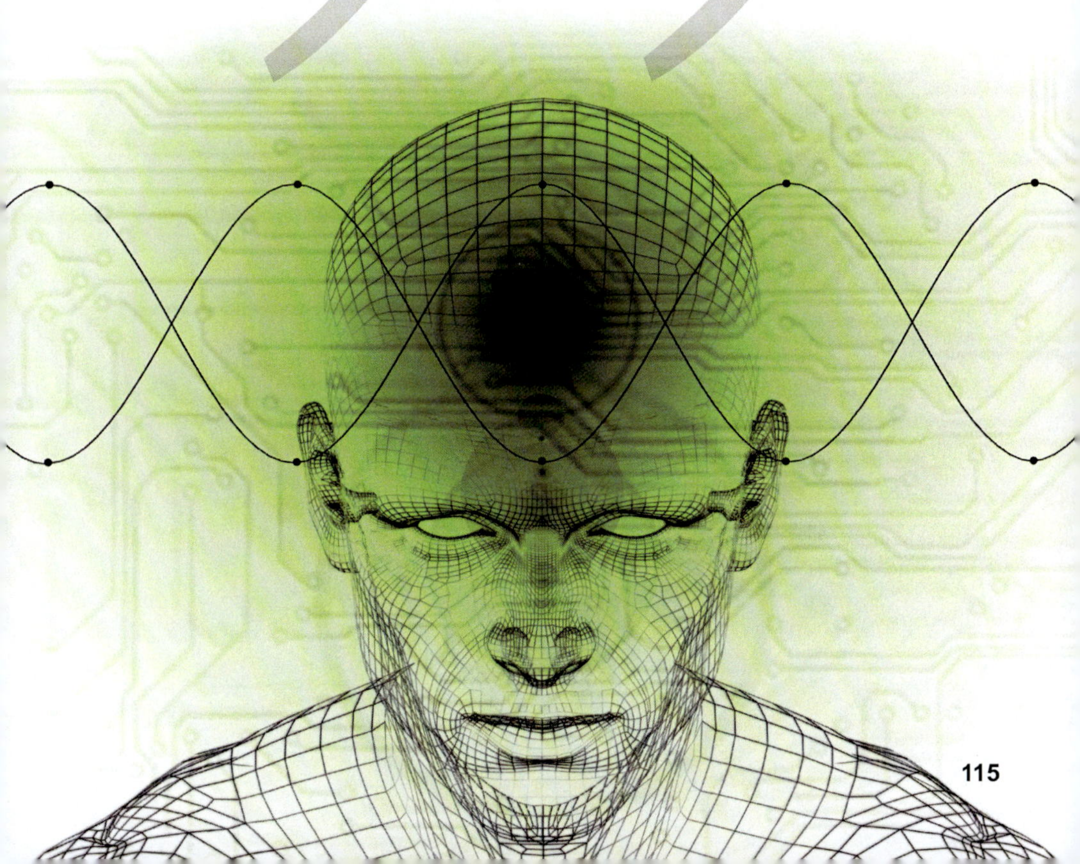

5.3.f. X-factor-1-2-3

The term "X-factor" describes the angular ratio of hip to shoulder axis in the backswing.

The ideal position of the shoulder at the end of the backswing is almost 90 degrees in relation to the ball-target line, while a rotation of less than 45 degrees is to be regarded as optimal for the hip in this connection.

These standards are also incontrovertible from a biomechanical standpoint – apart from the fact that the player inevitably loses balance in the backswing with the classic swing technique.

But the ratio of the angular position of the hip and shoulder axis is not only an important indication of the swing performance and the evaluation whether the swing is implemented physiologically – i.e. compatible with the body and joints – in the backswing, but also in subsequent swing phases.

Crucial moments of consideration in this connection are the moment of ball impact and the finish position.

X-factor-1

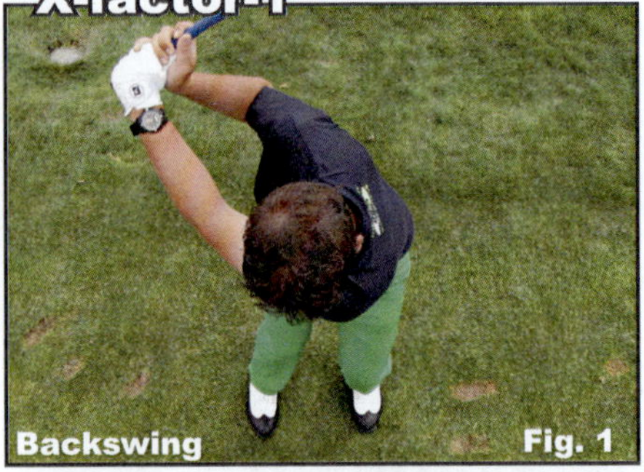

Backswing Fig. 1

aktive X-factor-2

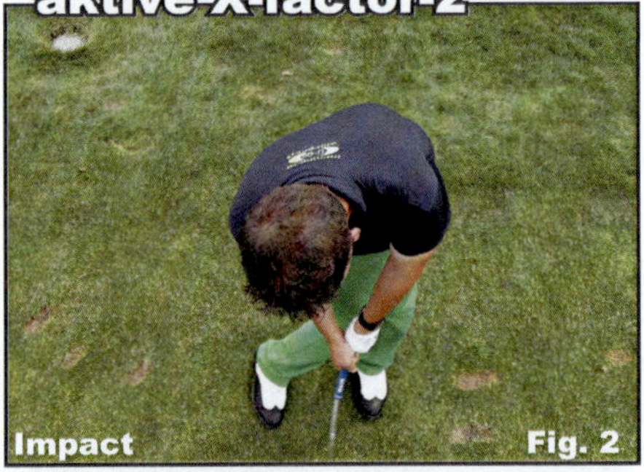

Impact Fig. 2

X-factor-3

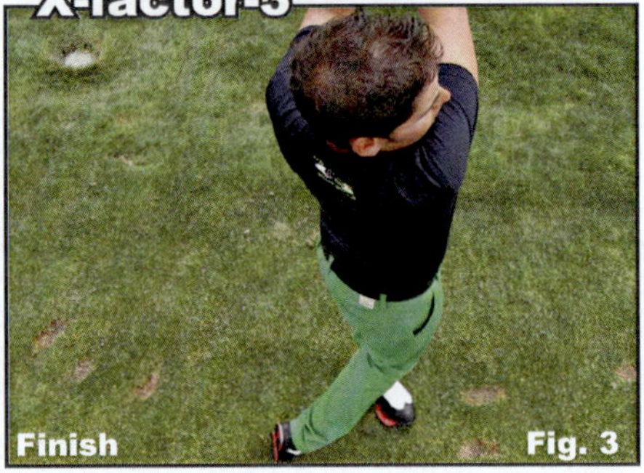

Finish Fig. 3

To that effect, I have expanded the known X-factor (backswing) by the X-factor 2 at the moment of impact and the X-factor 3 in the finish position and have created the FREE-RELEASE® X-factor-1-2-3 from this.

X-factor 2 refers to the pelvis-shoulder ratio at the moment of impact.

The following three stages are to be differentiated with regard to the pelvis at the moment of ball impact:

1. Negative X-factor-2: the hip is not turned and is in a neutral position (90 degrees towards the target, as in the setup).

2. Passive anticipatory X-factor-2: the pelvis is turned, but without active and controlled legwork.

3. Aktive X-factor-2: the hip is dynamically turned through use of active legwork (big toe joint). The ideal position lies at 67.5 degrees if the backswing angle of the hip is defined as the ideal position of 45 degrees. *(as 'zero angle'; see Fig 2)*

The swing sequence from golf Pro Angel Cabrera was pictured in the American magazine Golf Digest in 2010. There it is clearly discernible that Angel's hip at the moment of impact is in the same position as during setup.

The ideal value of the active X-factor-2 as defined by me is given with a hip rotation of approx. 67.5 degrees towards the target.

"At any level of performance there is approx. 20% unused potential which any golfer can harness to improve their performance through my method."

Frank Drollinger

5.4. Synchronize the backswing

The backswing is the foundation of all swing quality. It is important in this connection to synchronize the following aspects which come into play in terms of motion:

- **Balance**
- **Arms**
- **Hips**
- **Shoulders**

The arms are "thrust" with stable backs of hands towards the right thigh. The wrists only bend from this position. Hips and shoulders turn at the same time.

The result of this dynamic thrust rotation motion of the arms – synchronized with the hips and shoulders – is a "positioning" of the left upper arm on the torso.

Many golfers 'overwind' the pelvis by more than 45 degrees in

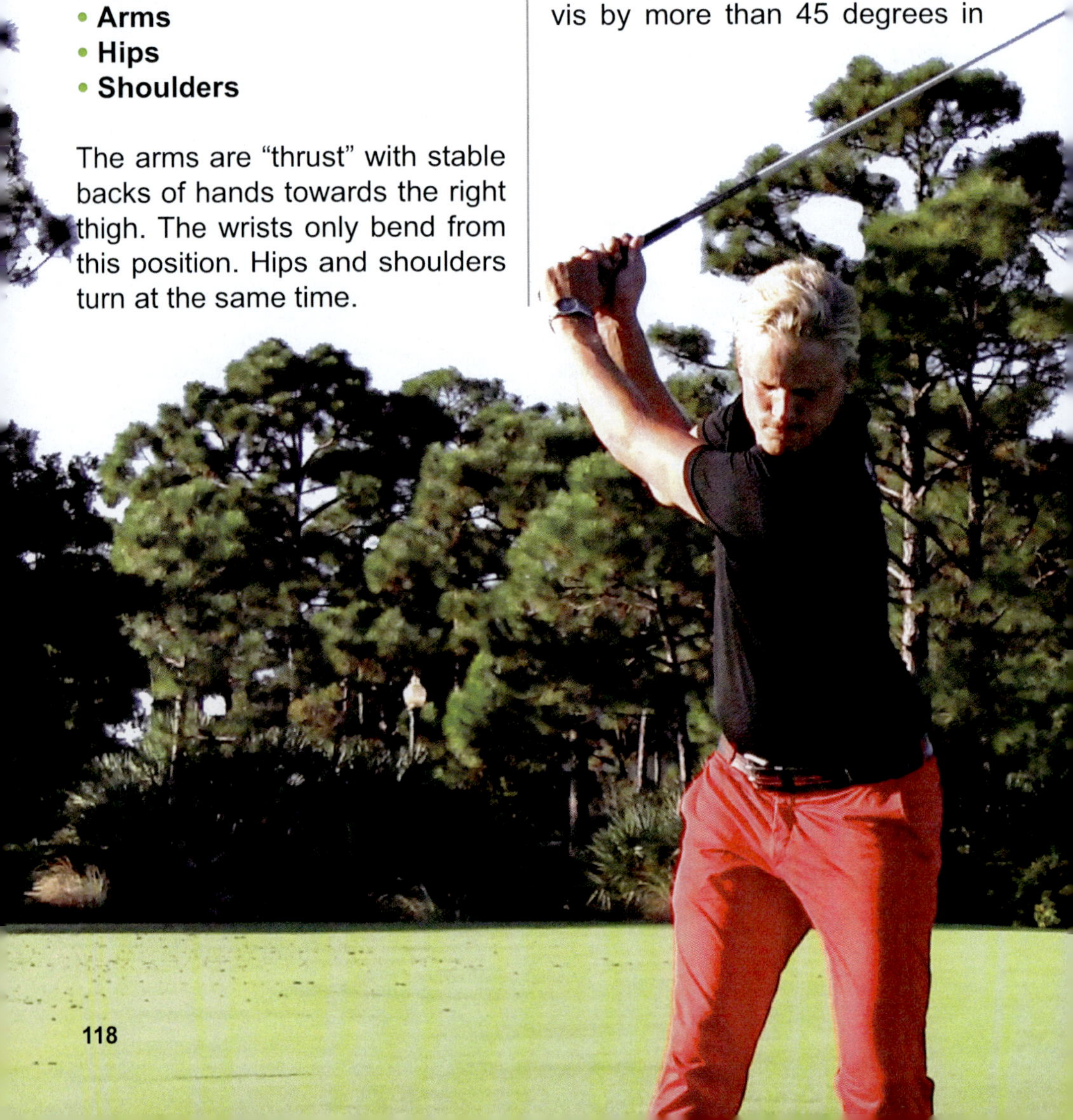

the backswing. This generates an imbalance. The shoulder may turn by up to 90 degrees. The backswing should be executed very slowly in order to keep the body's center of gravity and balance stable.

"Balance in the setup and backswing is the prerequisite for activating the large muscle groups of the right leg."

Frank Drollinger

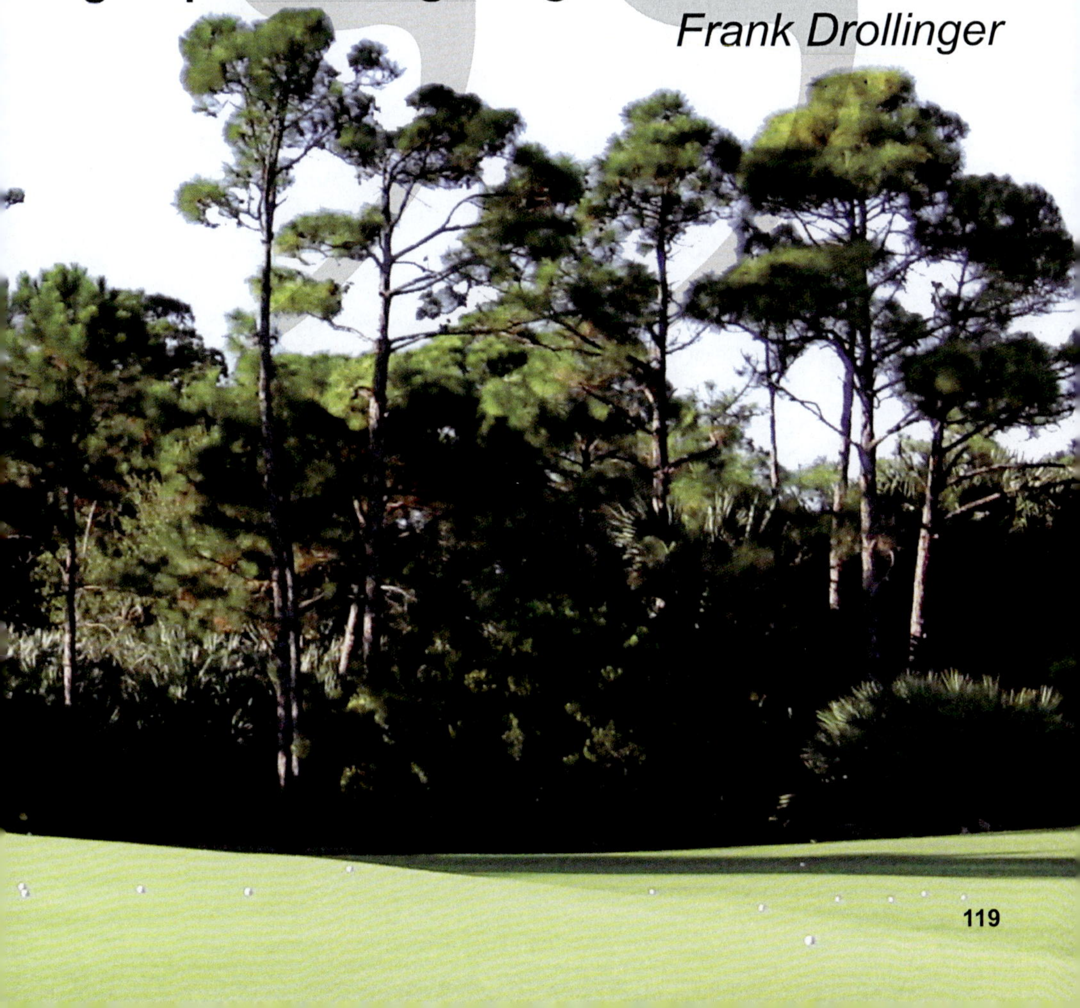

6. Golf & Olympics

From the viewpoint of sports medicine the Olympic Games are the best thing that could happen to golf.

The sport is enriched by a new quality, at least according to the rules: "...we have to do everything to reduce the risk of injuries....," hence sports medical research must be supported and not prevented.

Over the last 100 years the associations believed they could govern from an ivory tower and ignore everything that they did not like. The associations believe they can claim all benefits generated by the Olympic Games; however, the relevant obligations are still of no interest. I was told in St. Andrews by the R&A that golf will not be an Olympic discipline until 2016.

When I responded that according to the application regulations of the IOC, associations have to impose an obligation on their athletes prior to applying for the Olympic Games to adhere to the Olympic obligations, the surprise was great that I had delved so deep into the intricacies of the Olympic Games and golf.

The shocking finding in 2012 with regard to the Olympic Games and golf is that none of the top associations operates health management, publishes statistics on injuries, conducts sports science and sports medical research in order to reduce the injury rate.

There are even attempts to defend this backward status in full awareness that golfers therefore suffer injuries.

A paradox situation:
Dr. Digel, until 2012 the leading scientific expert within the German golf association DGV, co-author of an excellent book on the issue of health in high-performance sports that received state financial support, is not permitted to implement the more detailed demands that however conflict with those of the Medical Commission within the German association.

This behavior has been labeled as being "Amish" and "reactionary" by a sports sociologist. This may sound amusing, but it concerns the health of golfing children, adults, seniors and Tour players – and nobody should handle health in a negligent or intentionally harmful manner. The definition of intentional in this context includes conduct where the aversion of risk is ignored or prevented.

Many people, lawyers and sports sociologists with whom I have discussed the militant refusal to install functioning and sustainable health management within the associations have reported that the cause of this conduct must lie in the fact that decision-makers have been directly or indirectly bribed, or made compliant by advertising deals. When reviewing these considerations we established that almost all important national associations have corresponding advertising contracts. At the national level the decision-makers on the boards even have personal advertising contracts. For example, within the PGA Germany the 2012 president has contracts with an equipment company.

How can a methodically and sports medically objective decision then be made against a sponsor whose shoe sole system results in 15 times more torsional strain being placed on the golfer than do modern systems? The result of this system is that those representing its interests before the IGF are not impartial. For example, the German golf association DGV has advertising contracts with an equipment company; hence the representative sent to the IGF is not impartial.

I believe that the associations fail to analyze the consequences of contracts with equipment companies and advertising contracts.

Likewise, I believe that national associations follow international associations without considering the consequences.

I therefore demand:

1. that no decision-makers or board members of an association, or the association itself, be permitted to enter into advertising or equipment contracts or other business relationships with industrial enterprises in the field of golf.

2. that all national associations introduce a health passport for their athletes, who have to be looked after by a "GOLF-MEDICAL-COACH".

Overuse biomechanics

Overuse biomechanics that lead to injuries can no longer be considered good. Sports medical overuse is caused by "material fatigue" after long-term movements affect the joints, ligaments and tendons, intervertebral disks, bones, cartilage etc.

Golfers can only protect themselves against overuse biomechanics if there are biomechanical alternatives such as the FREE-RELEASE-Method® I developed and the "Turning Shoe."

For golfers of all ages **overuse means** that our joints, bones, ligaments and tendons, intervertebral disks, cartilage etc. are not constructed to perform the golf swing without damage occurring.

However, **overuse biomechanics also means** that movements are not synchronized. Where the legwork is passive, the upper body moves faster than the hips can follow. Or in the case of Rory McIlroy, the hips are accelerated by rapid rotation via the abdominal muscles.

Our bodies are not built for such long-term strain. **The result is injury.**

Since I have developed "Natural Motion Biomechanics" in the FREE-RELEASE-Method®, we are talking about avoidable injuries.

Due to the Olympic Games and their high-culture structures, the top associations would be in a position to exclude this risk and to take action to rectify the sports medical deficits in relation to other top associations.

This is what all other Olympic associations are doing. Examples and success stories are the helmet in ski sports. Nowadays all children wear helmets. It is irresponsible to expose the cartilage of children in particular to such negligent health risks where there are alternatives such as the Turning Shoe which do not affect the golf swing at all. The golf ball has been struck by the club face by the time the Turning Shoe unfolds its effect. **As a result the torsional strain is reduced by the measurable factor of 15**.

Golf Rule 14.3:
The Rules are unequivocal: According to Rule 14.3, "the player must not use any artificial device or unusual equipment ..., or use any equipment in an unusual manner ... that might assist him in making a stroke or in his play." This means that the player is unable to influence the flight of the ball after the moment of impact.

I have had long debates with the R&A and the USGA on this topic. I commissioned an expert opinion to be prepared by a physicist. A ball that has been struck cannot then be influenced by the player, the club, clothing, caps or shoes.

Health benefits arising <u>after</u> the moment of impact do not influence the golf swing.

I am even assuming that all shoe sole systems other than the Turning Shoe are not in line with the Rules since they exacerbate the risk of injury and hence should be banned under the Rules of Golf.

Exception 1:
This exception was introduced in 2007 on the basis of my work. At the time a product with a "medical reason" for using it was in principle permitted. Nowadays this has been modified so that there has to be a "medical condition." Here again, the Rules have been structured against the IOC regulations on health protection and prevention.

It was not clear to the R&A and the USGA that the "Turning Shoe" is a product with health benefits that do not arise until after the moment of impact.

7. Requirements for associations, organizations & functionaries

1. I call for the implementation of a functional system to protect the health of golfing children, adults, senior citizens, and top athletes.

2. I call for the implementation of the Rules of Golf — that golfers may not injure other golfers and consequently may also not injure themselves.

3. I demand that everything be done to reduce the risk of injury among golfers.

4. I call for implementation of the IOC Charter as well as the IOC Medical Code and the WADA Charter. I ask every individual golfer to help make sure that these requirements are implemented and adhered to.

I ask every individual golfer to help make sure that these requirements will be implemented and adhered to.

Frank Drollinger

8. Sports medical and kinematic results

I have initiated or personally implemented the following sports medicine and kinematic research projects (see below). A majority of related documents are available for free download at:

www.free-release.com

a) **2005:** University of Tübingen kinematic study on the influence of force by conventional golf shoe sole systems and the naturally turning "FREE-RELEASE®" sole system

b) **2005:** Electromyographic studies for comparison of muscular activity with conventional golf shoe sole systems and the naturally turning "FREE-RELEASE®" sole system

c) **2007:** University of Tübingen study pertaining to X-factor-1 and 3, the angular position of the hip and shoulder with conventional golf shoe sole systems and the naturally turning "FREE-RELEASE®" sole system

d) **2008:** Case studies conducted by Dr. Achim Rist from the Rennbahnklinik Basel (Swiss Olympic Medical Center) on the reduction of pain by conventional golf shoe sole systems and the naturally turning "FREE-RELEASE®" sole system

e) **2004 bis 2011:** Field trial with 5,000 golfers on the X-factor 1-2-3 angular position

"What we can learn from Formula 1 competition is the professionalism required to increase the likelihood of victory. This is exactly what we provide for recreational and professional golfers at the Golf-Biomechanic-Academy FREE-RELEASE®."

Frank Drollinger

Are Golfers Unscrupulous and Reactionary?

In my view: No. There are a small number of association officials and individuals who are harming the repute and credibility of the sport and who are not acting for the benefit of the overriding majority of golfers, who as in other sports want functional health management!

Examples:

"Presently we do not have time to attend to the health protection of golfers and of golfing children."
Alexander Klose, board member, Deutscher Golfer Verband, May 2012

„I have no idea about the sport of golf. I am not permitted to implement health management within the Deutscher Golf Verband."
Dr. Helmut Digel, scientific director, Deutscher Golf Verband

"Do we have to implement the obligations arising from the IOC Charta?"
Dr. Steve Otto, R & A, December 2011

"I am not in favour of golf becoming an Olympic sport."
Carter Ritch, USGA, January 2012 (At least Carter is honest and understands that the Olympic Games give rise to obligations as well as benefits)

"Does the R&A have contractual relations with the IOC?"
Dr. Steve Otto, R&A, December 2011 (R&A successfully applied to become an Olympic sports discipline, the IOC selected golf as an Olympic sports discipline. As a result and in accordance with the intentions of the participants, an agreement was brought about.)

"Golf is not an Olympic discipline until 2016. We do not have to take action today, and definitely do not have to implement the IOC Charta."
Dr. Steve Otto, R&A, December 2011 (The IOC Charta has to be implemented as of the application date, i.e. as of 2008, by every organized golfer, this means e.g. that the risk of injury has to be minimized.)

"The ball can be influenced by the player even after it has been hit."
Dr. Steve Otto, R&A, January 2012
(physically impossible, Dr. Ing., Dipl. Phys. Johannes Bertsch, 2012)

"First of all, a golfer has to suffer an injury. We are not interested in preventive health protection."
Dick Rugge, USGA (this attitude conflicts with the Rules of Golf, the spirit of the game, the IOC Charta, the WADA Charta and the ideals of the United Nations to further social progress in the sport of golf)

"We write the Rules and are not responsible for protecting golfers' health."
David Rickmann, R&A (Like the R&A, the USGA is a member of the IGF, which has undertaken to place an obligation on all associations to implement health protection. The IGF president is also the president of the R&A and wrote the introductory speech for the Olympic Games application.)

"I am familiar with the Olympic Charta – you're right, we have to do something – however, at the present time we do not want to address the possibilities of protecting the health of golfers."
Antony Scanlon, IGF

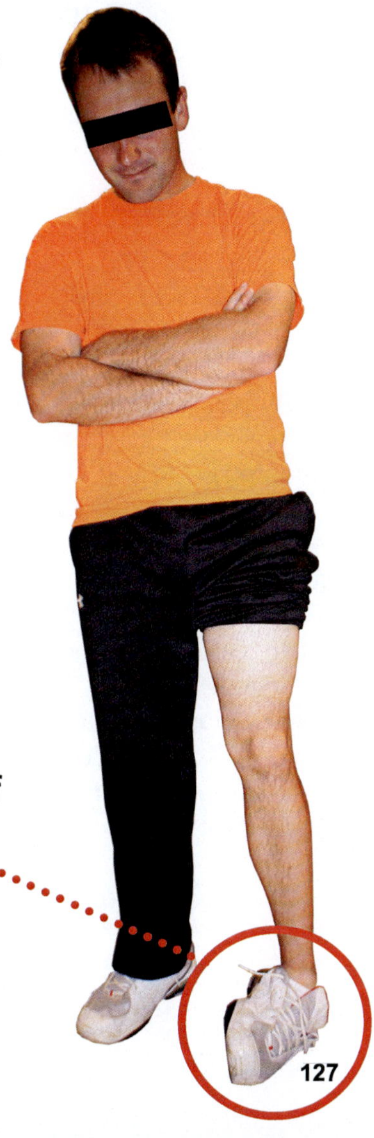

Consequences of many years of over-use biomechanics

Image shows an ex-European Tour player (24 years old – Diagnosis: chronic supination of the ankle joint)

Closing words

Dear Golfer,

I hope that reading this textbook has helped you to understand why the Golf-Active-Method FREE-RELEASE® is clearly superior to the conventional swing model according to Ben Hogan.

I cannot express often enough that in his era Ben Hogan was the greatest golf player and "teacher" for me.

I would like to pay homage to him.

Surely you will agree with me that in consideration of performance advantage and progressive biomechanics as well as in terms of sports medicine it is only logical that the Golf-Active-Method FREE-RELEASE® is the new control technique among golf swing methods. According to the current state of biomechanics, sports science and sports medicine, there is no better swing method than GAM FREE-RELEASE®.

I can assure you that with the Golf-Active-Method FREE-RELEASE® your advantage will not suffer a loss in the future — **because optimal biomechanics leave very little leeway for further improvements.**

Nobody – and last of all the top elite and professional players – can take the liberty of doing without medium-term methodical competitive advantages. Especially not the trainers of Tour players! That is why sooner or later all players, pros as well as amateur golfers, will swing according to my method.

And in view of a player's health, trainers and sports functionaries will learn that the principle of "Safety First" for professional golfers also represents a particular question with regard to sustainable career development and securing a livelihood.

The regulatory foundation of golf – the principle of the "spirit of the game" anchored in the Rules of

Golf, the IOC Charter and the provisions of WADA – calls for the best possible protection of the golfer's health. The Rules of Golf thereby make a plea for the application of GAM FREE-RELEASE® by every golfer and a departure in the educational and teaching system from old swing models.

It astonishes me how in some places clever and capable representatives of the educational system and functionaries quite doggedly – and in a reactionary manner – want to cling to an admittedly non-physiological and unhealthy golf swing motion. At this juncture, please ask yourself whether these individuals are free from advertising agreements and consequently act inhumanely at your "expense".

As an advocate of better health and injury protection in golf I sometimes feel like Robin Hood — a fighter with an honorable cause for the benefit of the entire golfing community. It is a good feeling!

I wish that all recalcitrant stak holders in golf return to the essentials – the athlete's health and fun in the game – and see the light:

GAM FREE-RELEASE® is the best, healthiest and most efficient golf swing method worldwide.

Do not believe anybody when it comes to the choice of your golf swing method, not even me! Instead, trust performance measurements and the scientific findings of biomechanical and sports medicine research efforts.

In future, those who want to be competitive in golf and comply with the Rules of Golf and the International Olympic Committee cannot avoid the overall system of GAM FREE-RELEASE®.

If the reading matter of this textbook has piqued your interest in meeting me personally, I would be

"90% of Tour players are dissatisfied with their swing, i.e. they sense that it could be even better. I can enable this improvement to Tour players and amateurs!"

Frank Drollinger

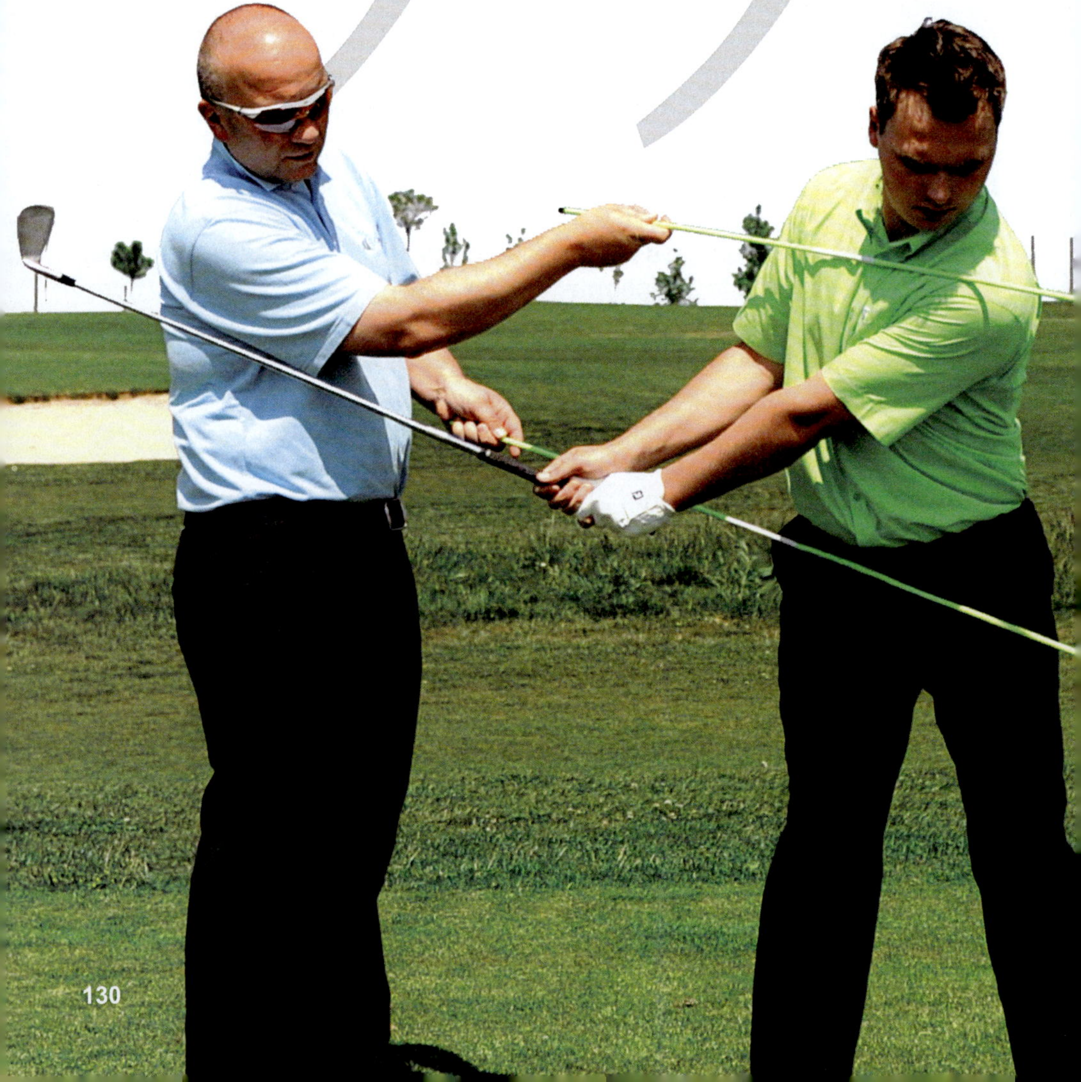

happy to welcome you as a participant of an advanced training course at our training center.
(overview of courses: **www.golf-active-method.com**)

Stay healthy and hearty!

Have fun playing!
Best regards,

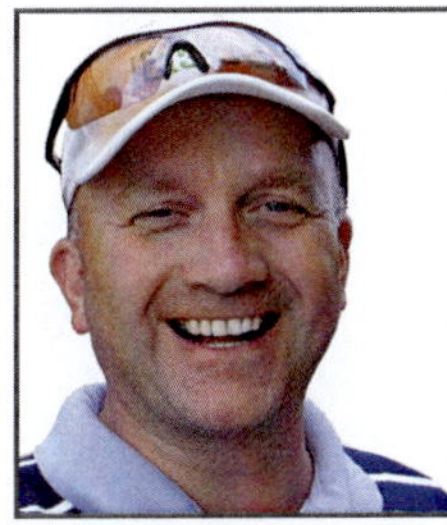

Yours, Frank Drollinger
Developer of FREE-RELEASE® system

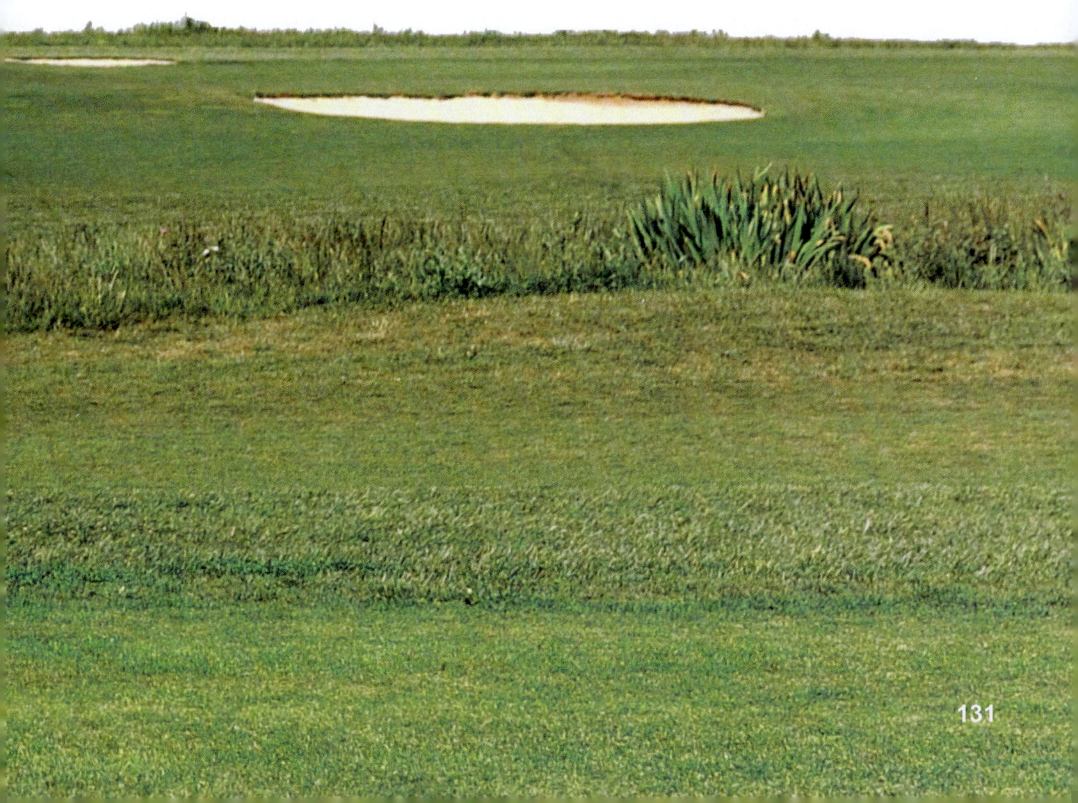

Expressions of thanks

People who we would particularly like to thank

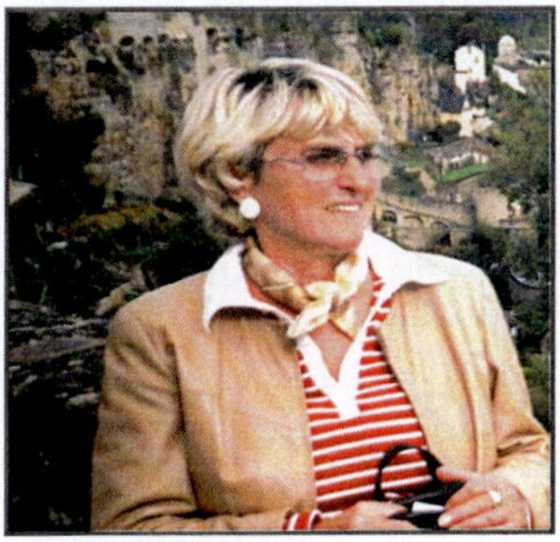

Heidi Sager †24.08.2009

My mother-in-law, source of inspiration for the development of the Turning Shoe!

She will always be remembered reverently by me and the United Golfers family.

Thank you!

The author

Frank Drollinger has analyzed and compared the motion of the golf swing for 23 years, and has also measured and analyzed kinematic and sports medicine data together with research partners in the fields of sports science and sports medicine for his book "GOLF: THE NEW TESTAMENT".

In this connection he gained a thorough knowledge of the unhealthy golf swing problem, and was the only person in the sports field that was able to establish motional as well as technically functional solutions for the main injury phenomena.

In a similar vein to his "method colleague", the great Ben Hogan, his driving force was dissatisfaction with his own golf swing method. If this driving force with Ben Hogan was the aspect of performance, with our author it was pain in the ankle and knee joints, pelvis and spine, which was caused by golf. Drollinger discovered that sustainable performance capability always leads by means of natural and consequently healthy kinematics.

His academic education, a diploma degree in the areas of sociology, psychology, actual state analyses, problem solving, solution finding, determination of qualified decision presentations, a 15-year biomechanical training period in kinematics and training as a consultant – as well as his self-practiced sports such as judo, handball, track and field athletics, alpine and Nordic skiing – were also responsible for the fact that the author is convinced that a team of experts is necessary to achieve top results.

For Drollinger it brings great joy that in spite of all the years of research and development, his efforts have brought about something very positive for the golfing world, golf athletes, golfing children, physicians, physiotherapists, trainers and organizations.

Starting from a non-physiological golf swing motion – which led and still leads to injuries among millions of golfers – he was able to create a healthy motion whose side effect enables a significant performance improvement, facilitation of motion and controllable repeatability.

In his function as Head Pro, Drollinger teaches golf biomechanics & health and measurable golf performance improvement for individual students as well as groups at his Golf-Biomechanic-Academy FREE-RELEASE® in Birkenfeld / Pforzheim (Germany) and in Orlando, Florida.

Drollinger is a vegetarian, impartial and sympathizes with Buddhism. The author preferably spends his very sparse free time together with his wife Andrea and friends while golfing, skiing or cooking.

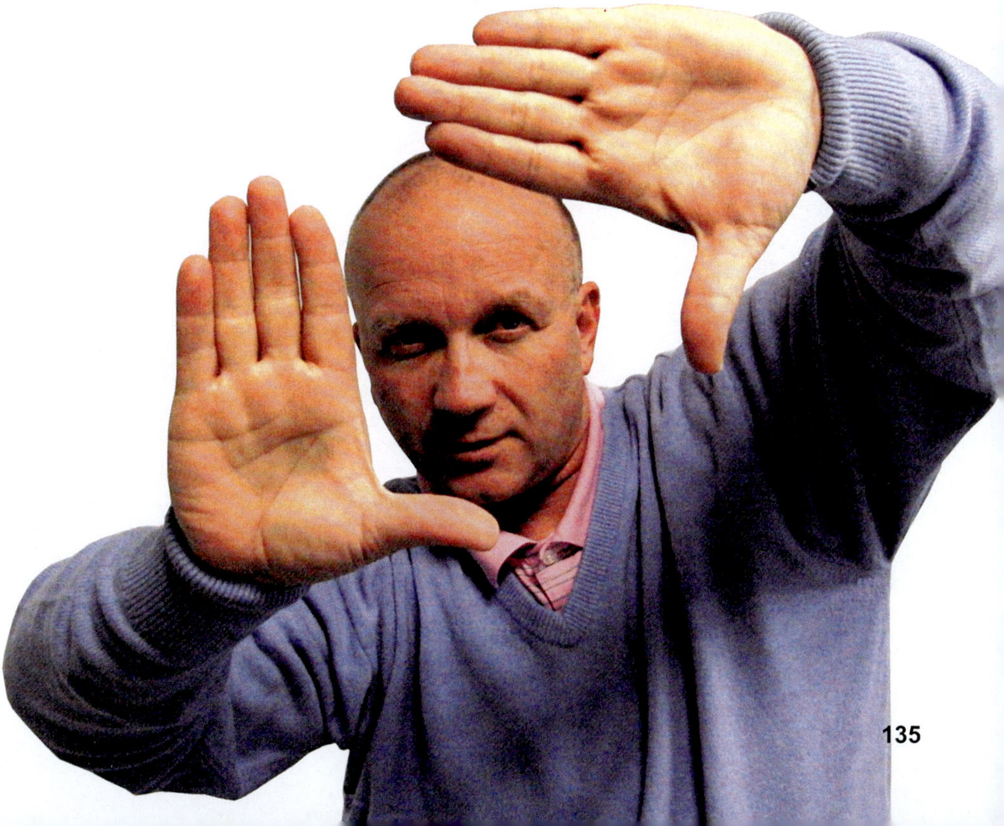

Glossary

A

Anticipation: Describes in sports science the mental and active anticipation of a future target-oriented sequence of movements.

B

Balance, vertical and horizontal:
Measurable balance; in the Golf-Active-Method FREE-RELEASE® we speak of set-up balance and backswing balance.

Balance Check (FREE-RELEASE®): With this test the angle positions of the hips and shoulder positions are established during the phases X-Factor-1 (final position in backswing), X-Factor-2 (ball impact) and X-Factor-3 (finish). X-Factor-1: hips -45 degrees, shoulders -90 degrees; X-Factor-2: hips +22.5 degrees, shoulders +22.5 degrees; X-Factor-3: hips +90 degrees, shoulders +90-105 degrees; these ideal measurements cannot be achieved with the Ben Hogan method.

Body's center of gravity:
Located approx. 5 cm behind the navel. The less it moves prior to ball impact, the larter the chance of achieving repeatable ball impact quality.

C

Core: Body's center of gravity. Should be as fixated as possible in a golfer during the set-up and backswing phases in order to render the stroke repeatable.

D

Doppler radar measurements:
Enables precise measurement of carry and overall length, clubhead and ball speed. (see also Smash7)

Double pendulum swing:
For 50 years the standardized golf swing method developed by Ben Hogan. With this method the arms and body each form a pendulum, hence the term double pendulum swing.

Dynamic axes parallelism: ensures that eyes, head, shoulder, pelvis, knees and feet axis stand at the same 90 degree angle in the direction of the target when the ball is teed off.

F

FREE-RELEASE®: Swing the club without encountering resistence in the body.

H

Hypermobile body's center of gravity:
Located approx. 5 cm behind the navel, should be fixated insofar as possible until ball impact. Prerequisite in order to be able to achieve repeatable ball impact quality.

L

Legwork, active: Triggered by the right big toe joint; objective: to accelerate the hips with the large muscle groups such as gluteal, upper and lower thighs as well as the foot towards the ball impact as fast as possible in order to improve the transfer of energy, and up to the finish (90 degrees) in order to reduce torsion in the spine.

Legwork, passive: Owing to the shift of weight on the backswing (Ben Hogan method), the leg muscles are mostly blocked so that active legwork is not possible. Consequences: the hips are torn towards the target in an uncontrolled manner by the diagonal abdominal muscles.

N

Natural Motion Biomechanics:
Describes a theory of movement which, contrary to over-use biomechanics, significantly reduces torsional and shearing forces etc. Includes in golf sport the FREE-RELEASE-Method® developed by Frank Drollinger.

O

Overuse-Biomechanics:
Describes theories of movement which cause injuries in the short, medium and long terms through torsional strain, shearing forces, friction, friction heat, vibrations and pressure caused by movement. All golf swing theories with passive legwork, no balance in set-up and backswing phases, and a hypermobile center of gravity during the set-up phase until ball impact, are covered by this description. These theories are not suitable for functional health management.

R

Rotational impulse: Movement triggered in the back foot, i.e. the right foot is propelled towards the target dynamically and in a controlled manner through a strong impulse so that the hips can be accelerated in a controlled manner by approx. 67.5 degrees until ball impact.

S

Smash7: Figure determined by radar measurement devices and kinematics. Includes according to Frank Drollinger the ball and clubhead speed, lateral deviation in ball flight, to the left or to the right, spin factor, distance, duration of flight, height of flight, impact angle ball/clubface, and kinematically determined torque.

Spin-Factor: Number of ball rotations towards the target and lateral.

T

Torque: Newton; a measured torque is an expression of the forces affecting the golfer.

Torsional moment: A torsional moment measured in Newton meters releases the influence of force on the golfer here.

X

X-Factor-1: Angle position of pelvis and shoulders in final backswing position.

X-Factor-2: Angle position of pelvis and shoulders at the moment of ball impact.

X-Factor-3: Angle position of pelvis and shoulders in finish position.

Bibliography

- Blatt, M. E. : A Survey of Golf Injuries in Amateur Golfers. In: British Journal of Sports Medicine Nr. 26 (1): 1992, S.63-65.
- Boldt, F. / Wolff, R.: Sportmedizinische Aspekte des Golfsports. In: Deutsches Ärzteblatt Nr. 98 (37): 2001, S. 1886-1889.
- Bosch, H.-C.: Sportmedizinisches Gutachten zum Thema: Gegenüberstellung gesundheitlicher Auswikungen und Risikoeinschätzung des „Turning Shoes" im Vergleich zu herkömmlichen Schuhsohlensystemen im Golfsport. Stockach: 2012.
- Castro, W. H. M. / Schilgen, M.: Kreuzschmerzen. Ursachen, Behandlung, Vorbeugung. Gütersloh: 2003.
- Cochran, A. J. / Stobbs, J.: Search for the Perfect Swing. Chicago: 1999.
- Göhner, U.: Bewegungslehre des Sports (Teil 1). Schorndorf: 1992.
- Golf Digest: Golfer Health Study 2006, The Golf Digest Publications Research Resource Center: 2006.
- Gosheger, G. u.a.: Injuries and Overuse Syndromes in Golf. In: The American Journal of Sports Medicine Nr. 31: 2003, S. 438-443.
- Gregori, A. C. P.: Tibial Stress Fractures in Two Professional Golfers. In: Journal of Bone & Joint Surgery [British Vol.] Nr. 76B: 1994, S. 157-158.
- Guten, G. N.: Knee Injuries in Golf. In: Clinical Journal of Sports Medicine Nr. 15 (1): 1996, S. 111-128.
- Hogan, B.: Der Golfschwung. Stuttgart: 1957.
- Hosea, T. / Gatt, C. / Gertner, E.: Biomechanic Analysis of the Golfer's Back. In: Stover, C. u.a. (Hg.): Feeling Up to Par: Medicine from Tee to Green. Philadelphia: 1994, S. 97-108.
- Lauterburg, M.: Der Golfschwung, der Ihren Rücken schont. In: Drive Nr. 9: 2003, S. 54-55.
- Letzelter, H.: Golftechniken - Wieso, weshalb, warum? Eine Trainings- und Bewegungslehre des Golfspiels. Münster: 2002.
- Pässler, H. H.: Knieverletzungen im Golf und deren Prophylaxe. In: ATOS news Nr. 15: 2010, S. 10-12.
- Rist, H. J. / Ulrich, M.: Case Report – Eine Innovation im Golfschuhbau von sportmedizinischer Bedeutung. Therapeutischer Einsatz an drei Fallbeispielen. In: Sport Orthopädie Traumatologie Nr. 26: 2010, S. 29-33.

- Rist, H. J.: Medizinisch sinnvoller Paradigmenwechsel im Golfschuhbau? In: ATOSnews Nr. 15: 2010, S. 13-16.
- Schiebl, F.: Forschungsbericht. Forschungsprojekt „D-Carver“. Tübingen: 2005.
- Schiebl, F.: Zusatzgutachten zum Forschungsprojekt „D-Carver“. Medizinisch-orthopädische Schlussfolgerungen zur Verwendung des FREE-RELEASE® Golfschuhs. Sindelfingen: 2007.
- Seaman, D.: A Review of Back Pain in Golfers. Etiology and Prevention. In: Sports Medicine Training and Rehabilitation Nr. 9: 2000, S. 169-188.
- Siebert, W.: Erster Erfahrungsbericht über den so genannten „Free-Release“-Golfschuh – Reduktion der Gelenk- und Wirbelsäulenbelastung beim Golfspiel. In: Orthopädische Praxis Nr. 43: 2007, S. 681-683.
- Thiel, A. / Mayer, J. / Digel, H.: Gesundheit im Spitzensport – eine sozialwissenschaftliche Analyse. Schorndorf. 2010.
- Wank, V.: Biomechanical Analysis of the Motion Kinematics of Selected Body Axes During the Golf Swing When Using a Normal Golf Shoe or a Free-Release Golf Shoe Developed by United Golfers. Tübingen: 2007.